OPHTHALMIC DRUG DELIVERY
BIOPHARMACEUTICAL, TECHNOLOGICAL AND CLINICAL ASPECTS

OPHTHALMIC DRUG DELIVERY

BIOPHARMACEUTICAL, TECHNOLOGICAL AND CLINICAL ASPECTS

Edited by

M.F. Saettone
Istituto di Chimica Farmaceutica
dell'Università di Pisa, Italy

M. Bucci
Clinica Oculistica,
Università dell'Aquila, Italy

P. Speiser
Pharmazeutisches Institut ETHZ,
Zurich, Switzerland

FIDIA
RESEARCH
SERIES

Volume 11

Springer Science+Business Media, LLC

FIDIA RESEARCH SERIES

An open-end series of publications on international biomedical research, with special emphasis on the neurosciences, published by LIVIANA Press, Padova, Italy, in cooperation with FIDIA Research Labs, Abano Terme, Italy.

The series will be devoted to advances in basic and clinical research in the neurosciences and other fields.

The aim of the series is the rapid and worldwide dissemination of up-to-date, interdisciplinary data as presented at selected international scientific meetings and study groups.

Each volume is published under the editorial responsibility of scientists chosen by organizing committees of the meetings on the basis of their active involvement in the research of the field concerned.

Originally published by Springer-Verlag Berlin Heidelberg New York Tokyo in 1987
MyCopy version of the original edition 1987

DOI 10.1007/978-1-4757-4175-9

LIVIANA Editrice S.p.A. - via Luigi Dottesio 1, 35138, Padova, Italy.
www.springer.com/mycopy

CONTENTS

PREFACE

This book contains the proceedings of the International Symposium on Ophthalmic Drug Delivery, which was held in Pisa in October 1986. Topical ophthalmic therapy is a matter of interest to specialists from different fields (medical, pharmaceutical, chemical, technological, etc.), who, unfortunately, have a tendency to meet separately, thus limiting a diffusion of knowledge, ideas and experience that would greatly favour the overall progress in this area of research.

The Symposium, for the first time in Europe, provided the opportunity for specialists from different disciplines and from different countries to meet, to discuss and to share their experience. This multidisciplinary approach is reflected in the wide variety of topics that appear in the book. The papers are aimed at reviewing many of the complex, interrelated, medical pharmaceutical and technological facets of topical ophthalmic therapy. It is our hope that they may stimulate further thought in this fascinating field, and may provide possible guidelines for future research.

The editors wish to express their appreciation to the sponsors of the Symposium: Fidia Research Laboratories, whose generosity permitted the meeting to be held, and the Italian National Research Council (CNR, Progetto Finalizzato Chimica Fine e Secondaria) who gave its scientific tutorship. Thanks are also due to the other Symposium contributors, ACRAF SpA, Rome, and Allergan Italia SpA, Rome. The assistance, support and cooperation given before, during and after the Symposium by Dr. Patrizia Chetoni, Dr. Maria Tilde Torracca and Dr. Elena Parolini are also gratefully acknowledged.

Marco Fabrizio Saettone
Massimo Bucci

Pisa, June 1987

INTRODUCTION

These proceedings reflect the broad spectrum of topics which have been recently treated at an International Ophthalmic Symposium in Pisa, Italy. It represents the anatomic, physiologic, pharmaceutical, technological, pharmacodynamic and clinical current knowledge on ocular drug delivery. Special attention is paid to the recent formulative aspects, the methods of obtaining true controlled or real sustained release. Furthermore, the biological and chemical evaluation of topical ophthalmic vehicles containing natural or synthetic additives as polymers, latexes, nanoparticles and inserts are negotiated. Finally, the above mentioned aspects of novel dosage forms are discussed very frankly and demonstrate the titanic background the ocular specialists must have under control nowadays.

The topics of this Symposium were selected by a scientific committee piloted by Prof. M.F. Saettone (Pisa), successfully combining the formulation problems (Prof. Buri, Geneva) with the industrial queries (Prof. E. Chiellini, Pisa) and the biological-clinical aspects (Prof. G. Bucci, L'Aquila). We would like to express our appreciation to the invited speakers for conforming to the deadlines and delivering their manuscripts so promptly. This results in the opportunity to publish these proceedings shortly after the Congress so that every specialist interested and engaged in ophthalmic therapy and ocular drug formulation design may soon make himself familiar with the recent progress in the various fields.

P. Speiser

OCULAR ANATOMY AND PHYSIOLOGY: ITS RELEVANCE TO TRANSCORNEAL DRUG ABSORPTION AND TO VEHICLE EFFECTS

M. Peduzzi, A. Debbia and A. Monzani

Department of Ophthalmology
University of Modena, Italy

Owing to easy accessibility of the eyeball, topically applied drugs are widely employed in ophthalmology for both diagnostic and therapeutic purposes.

In spite of a variety of defense mechanisms which protect the eye from noxious substances in the environment (as the continuous secretion of tears which coats an impermeable surface epithelium), topical administration of drugs on the eye surface allows persistence of therapeutic levels of medications for clinically effective durations of time and minimizes unwanted collateral systemic effects, though these substances can rapidly spread to all parts of the body.

This paper reviews the current knowledge of the mechanisms by which structural and functional characteristics of the eye and its adnexa can interfere with intraocular penetration of topically applied drugs.

A number of techniques including transmission and scanning electron microscopy, specular microscopy, electrophysiological measurements and cell culture have recently provided valid tools for the study of functional morphology of ocular tissues and fluids in relation to drug penetration into the globe.

Many studies have been carried out in these last decades both in Europe and United States and it would be impossible here to consider all of them. However I would like to acknowledge this morning the pioneering work done by Dr. Maurice and his group in this field.

For didactic purposes we will consider step by step the various obstacles encountered by medications on their way from the outside to the inside of the eye.

The first impact is on the lacrimal film: the characteristics of tear distribution and flow greatly affect one of the most important factors involved in intraocular drug penetration, i.e. the contact time between the vehicle-drug complex and the ocular surface, which is defined as the area under the curve that relates drug concentration in the tear film to time.

Contact-time may be prolonged by means of various techniques, such as increased viscosity of drops or other engineered devices: however it is mainly influenced by the tear flow, which is known to be variable in different subjects and in different situations.

As a general rule, the rapid washout with drops instilled into the conjunctival sac leads to immediate loss of a great part of the drug.

In fact, the total volume of fluid the eye can hold being 10 μl, only about 20% of a drop delivered by commercial eye droppers (the volume of which is about 50 μl) can be retained by the eye.

Ophthalmic Drug Delivery. Biopharmaceutical, Technological and Clinical Aspects.
M.S. Saettone, G. Bucci, P. Speiser (eds.) Fidia Research Series, vol. 11, Liviana Press, Padova © 1987

Five minutes after administration, only 8% of the original 20% of the drop remains in the conjunctival sac, owing to rapid turnover rate of tears (16% per minute).
Additional loss of medication usually occurs since a faster turnover rate may result from reflex tearing caused by the irritation of the drop.
The composition of tears includes various substances such as proteins, electrolytes, vitamins, enzymes, glucose and others, which may play a role in the transfer of drugs to the cornea. For example, proteins derived from the secretory glands of the conjunctiva may bind drugs in the tear fluid, further reducing their effective concentration.
In normal conditions when the eye is open the lacrimal fluid is divided into three separate compartments: a) the precorneal film which covers the exposed cornea and conjunctiva; b) a mostly stagnant layer moistening the conjunctiva under the lids; c) the marginal tear strips along which the tear flow occurs.
The precorneal film in turn is composed of three layers: the superficial oily layer is primarily derived from the meibomian glands and restricts the evaporation of the underlying watery layer which is mostly produced by the lacrimal glands. The innermost mucoid layer is derived from the conjunctival globet cells and is effective in stabilizing the tear film.
During a blink the mucin layer is spread over the cornea, thus maintaining its normal wetting and producing a hydrophilic surface for the tear film.
Moreover the act of blinking, mixing the three compartments of the lacrimal fluid, leads to redistribution of substances dissolved in the precorneal film: for example a drug dissolved in a drop instilled into the conjunctival sac is mixed to some extent with the tear fluid, being diluted so that the concentration is quickly reduced to about one third of that in the original drop. Drug concentration has been shown to undergo a continual decline in a roughly exponential manner.
Drugs dissolved in the lacrimal film penetrate the globe almost exclusively through the cornea, most of the material which crosses the conjunctiva being rapidly lost to the blood stream, and only small portions diffusing through the limbal zone and the sclera. In fact the conjunctival epithelium acts as a barrier against penetration of substances under the conjunctiva, but it appears to be weaker than the corneal epithelium. When in the subconjunctival space, drugs are rapidly lost to the blood before having the possibility to penetrate into the deeper tissues. This could give reason for unpleasant systemic side effects sometimes occurring after instillation of drugs into the conjunctival sac, and for reduced therapeutic efficacy of topical medications in diseases affecting the back of the eye.
The cornea may act as a pathway, a barrier or a reservoir of drugs. Of the five layers in which the cornea is classically divided, only the sandwich consisting of the stromal connective tissue covered by epithelial and endothelial cellular layers is relevant to transcorneal drug penetration. The barrier is mainly represented by the epithelium, the reservoir by the stroma (particularly for hydrophilic substances), while the role of the endothelium is negligible for both aspects.

The epithelium and the endothelium, rich in lipids and cells, are mostly permeable to substances possessing a fat-soluble phase, while the stroma, characterized by relative acellularity and a high water content, is mostly permeable to substances possessing a water-soluble phase. Therefore, to be able to pass through the intact cornea, substances must be soluble in both fats and water, since purely water-soluble substances cannot penetrate the epithelium and purely fat-soluble substances cannot penetrate the stroma.
Epithelium occupies about 10% of total corneal thickness and is composed of five to six layers of cells, increasing to eight to ten at the corneal periphery.
Three groups of cells are usually identified in the epithelium: a single row of basal cells, an intermediate zone of two or three layers of polygonal cells (wing cells), and a couple of superficial layers of large , flattened cells, which are characteristically joined by tight junctions, and present surface microplicae and microvilli which could play a role in the retention of precorneal film. The barrier effect of corneal epithelium is mainly due to the presence of tight junctions, which probably represent the most difficult hurdle to penetration of ionic solutes.
In fact the dissociated ions such as Na^+ and Cl^- pass the cellular layers slowly through the paracellular pathways, like other ionized substances (as for example fluorescein).
The arrangement of superficial epithelial cells leads to an increase of the path distance, owing to flattening and overlapping of these cells, the large diameter of which allows relatively few intercellular spaces which open on the outer surface of the cornea.
Undissociate salts on the other hand are fat-soluble and can pass more rapidly trough cell membranes.
The fat solubility of a substance depends, among other factors, on its non-polar nature, i.e. on possessing an extremely symmetric atomic structure. These substances therefore penetrate more rapidly into the eye when the epithelium is intact than when it is disrupted or absent (the contrary, of course, occurring with water-soluble substances).
Surface active materials, some of which are used as ophthalmic preservatives, have been demonstrated to reduce the resistance of epithelial cells; however scanning electron microscopy has well documented the destructive effect of some of them, such as benzalkonium chloride, on the outermost cell layer.
The permeability of corneal epithelium to different substances varies considerably according to their dissociation , which is mainly dependent upon the hydrogen ion concentration (pH) of the solution in which they are dissolved.
As a general rule weak bases (various alkaloids and the majority of local anesthetics) increase their water solubility as they undergo dissociation; conversely they increase in lipid solubility with decreasing dissociation . These drugs in solutions can remain both in the dissociated and undissociate forms, thus possessing properties of both fat and water solubility. The undissociated fraction will be greater at higher pH values, and consequently the drug will increase in lipid solubility and readly penetrate the epithelium.

Moreover epithelial permeability has been shown to decrease in anoxic conditions, as can occur in patients using extended wear contact lenses.

Superficial cell layers have also been indicated as the major source of resistance in the epithelium by investigations of the electrical potential of the corneal surface with penetrating microelectrodes.

On their way toward the anterior chamber, and once passed the strong epithelial barrier , drugs meet with the stroma, composed almost entirely of collagenous lamellae, and constituting nine tenth of the thickness of the entire cornea. The stroma can be considered a comparatively open structure which allows diffusion of solutes having molecular weight below 500.000 in normal conditions, and even larger when oedematous. It can act as a barrier for very lipophilic substances which pass freely through the epithelium, while it is easily penetrated by hydrophilic solutes.

The stroma is in contact with the endothelium, which constitutes the innermost layer of the corneal sandwich.

The posterior surface of the cornea represents a weak barrier, the endothelium being about 200 times more permeable than the epithelium. The endothelium comprises a single layer of thin polygonal cells, and its permeability characteristics suggest that most of the penetration takes place through inert pores which could correspond to the intercellular spaces.

The endothelial layer is crossed by a passive flux of water toward the stroma, which has a tendency to swell, and by an active flux in opposite direction due to its active pump mechanism which controls corneal turgescence. However solutes diffuse freely across the endothelium, without being appreciably affected by either active or passive flux of water.

The endothelium represents the last obstacle to intraocular penetration of topically applied drugs, but a question could arise about what actually has reached the anterior chamber. In fact some drugs are known to be broken down by the tissues during intraocular penetration, so that not only the original compounds are found in the anterior chamber, but also their metabolites which in general are less active.

Therefore transcorneal penetration results in a rather remarkable decrease in concentration and efficacy of the drug originally instilled into the conjunctival sac.

Intrinsec permeability characteristics of corneo-conjunctival surface are basically not susceptible to modifications induced by therapeutic interventions; therefore we can act only on factors influencing the contact time, the phase solubility and the diffusion of the drug out of the vehicle, at the same time seeking a better knowledge of the interactions between these factors and the ocular structures. This actually appears to be the major goal of researchers and drug companies in order to optimize transcorneal penetration of medications.

SUGGESTED READINGS

Adler F.H.: Physiology of the eye, 4th edition, c.v. Mosby Co., St. Louis 1985, p. 42.

Burstein N.L.: Corneal citotoxicity of topically applied drugs, vehicles and preservatives. Survey of Ophthalmol., 25(1),15, 1980.

Doane M.D., Jensen A.D., Dohlman H.: Penetration routes of topically applied eye medications. Am. J. Ophthalmol. 85,383, 1978.

Ellis P.P., Smith D.L.: Handbook of ocular therapeutics and pharmacology, 4th edition. c.v. Mosby Co., St. Louis 1983, p. 3.

Gaster R.N., Leopold I.N.: Pharmacologic principles in the treatment of corneal disease. In: Biomedical Foundation of Ophthalmology, Duane T.D. and Jaeger E.A. Edts, Vol.III, Harper & Row Publishers, Philadelphia, 1982, p. 1.

Havener W.H.: Ocular pharmacology, c.v. Mosby Co., St. Louis 1974, p. 19.

Hogan M.J., Alvarado J.A., Weddel J.E.: Hystology of the human eye. An atlas and textbook. W.B. Saunders Co., Philadelphia 1971, p. 55.

Jakobieck F.A.: Ocular anatomy, embriology and teratology, Harper & Row Publishers, Philadelphia 1982, p. 153.

Klyce S.D.: Electrical profiles in the corneal epithelium. J. Physiol. 226,407, 1972.

Maurice D.M., Mishima S.: Ocular pharmacokinetics. In: Pharmacology of the Eye, M.L. Sears Ed., Springer Verlag 1984, p. 20.

Maurice D.M.: The cornea and sclera in: The Eye, 3rd Edition, Dawson H. Ed., Vol.1B, Academic Press Orlando (Florida), 1984.

Pfister R.R., Burstein N.: The effects of ophthalmic drugs, vehicles and preservatives on corneal epithelium: a scanning electron microscope study. Invest. Ophthalmol. 15,246, 1981.

Tonjum A.M., Green K.: The effect of benzalkonium chloride on the electropotential of the rabbit cornea. Acta Ophthalmol. 53,348, 1975.

Wine N.A., Gornall A.G., Basu P.K.: The ocular uptake of subconjunctivally injected C14 hydrocortisone. Am. J. Ophthalmol. 58,362, 1964.

FACTORS INFLUENCING THE RETENTION OF OPHTHALMIC SOLUTIONS ON THE EYE SURFACE

M.M. Van Ooteghem

Department of Pharmaceutical Sciences, University of Antwerp
Universiteitsplein 1, B-2610 Wilrijk, Belgium

The instillation of an ophthalmic solution generally initiates reflex tears and reflex blinking, which attempt to remove quickly the instilled solution from the eye surface. Reflex tears and reflex blinking are often elicited by different properties of the instilled solutions, such as the instilled volume, the osmolality, the pH and viscosity of the solution, and also by the physical and chemical properties of the drugs and the adjuvants present.

INTRODUCTION

The bioavailability of ophthalmic solutions containing drugs active on the eye surface or after resorption through the cornea increases with the retention time of the drug on the eye surface. Instilled eyedrops, however, are rapidly eliminated. Sorensen and Jensen (1979) registered the radioactivity remaining on the eye surface after the instillation of a suspension containing a radioactive tracer (Tc-99m). The radioactivity was reduced by two-thirds within two minutes and the tracer was completely eliminated after 15 minutes. The decay occurred in three steps: a very fast elimination during the two first minutes, followed by a rapid one between 2 and 5 minutes, and finally, a slow elimination 7 to 15 minutes after instillation were observed.

The elimination is due to the different defence mechanisms of the eye against foreign matter. The cornea and the conjunctiva are protected by tears and by the eyelids, which are responsible for the elimination of foreign matter, such as ophthalmic solutions. An increase in tear production or reflex tears and an increase in the blink rate or reflex blinking may be elicited by different stimuli, such as painful and irritating solutions.

The painful sensation and irritation are not the same for each preparation. Some eyedrops elicit more reflex tears and a higher reflex blinking than other collyria. These differences can be attributed to the different properties of the preparations and to their different administration procedures. The properties which may thus influence retention are: the instilled volume, the osmolality, the pH and the viscosity of the solutions as well as the properties of the drugs and the adjuvants.

In this paper the elimination processes and the preparation properties that may influence elimination are discussed.

Ophthalmic Drug Delivery. Biopharmaceutical, Technological and Clinical Aspects.
M.S. Saettone, G. Bucci, P. Speiser (eds.) Fidia Research Series, vol. 11, Liviana Press, Padova © 1987

TEARS

The eye is covered by a thin precorneal tear film, which is composed of three layers: a mucin, a water, and a lipid layer, and is formed by the basal tears. Tears are continuously secreted by different glands and by the goblet cells. The average secretion of basal tears is 1.2 µl/min (Mishima et al.,1966). The tears flow continuously over the surface of the cornea and conjunctiva, where a part of the water evaporates, while the remaining tears are drained by the puncti to the lacrimal sac.

Reflex tears are secreted under the influence of stimuli: the main and the accessory lobes of the lacrimal glands are responsible for these reflex tears. Only the watery layer of the precorneal film is increased, disturbing the precorneal film structure (Hawes and Ellis, 1985). The lipid layer would no longer act as a good barrier to prevent the evaporation of the water, and formation of "dry spots" may occur (Rolando and Refojo, 1983).

Reflex tears, which are evoked by sensory stimuli from the nerves ending in the cornea, are stimulated by an exposure of the eye to light, cold, wind, foreign bodies or irritating liquids such as ophthalmic solutions (Walsh and Hoyt, 1969a). An instillation of an irritant solution (e.g. 1 µl of a saturated potassium chloride solution) in the eye elicits reflex tearing after 30 to 40 seconds (Wright, 1985).

The volume of reflex tears, which is influenced by the irritating power of the instilled solution, varies from 3 µl/min to 300/400 µl min (Lamberts et al., 1979; Jordan and Baum, 1979; Jordan and Baum, 1980; Farris et al., 1981). The patient, however, is not always aware of the increased tear flow (Mishima, et al., 1966).

Reflex tears eliminate drugs from the eye surface more rapidly than basal tears. The decay of radioactivity observed by Sorensen and Jensen (1979), occurring from 2 to 5 minutes after instillation, is due to the secretion of reflex tears; the subsequent slow elimination is due to basal tears.

THE MOVEMENT OF THE EYELIDS

The upper eyelid moves mainly in a vertical direction over two-thirds of the eye surface. This downward motion appears to act as a "scraper", the surface of the cornea being cleaned and debris and foreign matter, such as ophthalmic preparations, being pushed into contact with the lower eyelid. The main motion of the lower eyelid is a horizontal translation in a nasal direction, sometimes as much as 4 or 6 mm. This action appears to move the tear fluid, incorporated debris, and foreign matter to the nasal corner of the lid junction, where the liquid exits via the puncti (Doane, 1979).

The tear film thickness is markedly affected by the force, the velocity and frequency of blinking. Rapid and forceful blinking squeezes lacrimal fluid out of the conjunctival sac and substantially increases the tear film thickness. A slow and weak blinking seems to decrease the thickness of the tear film (Benedetto, 1982; Benedetto et al., 1984).

The velocity of the eyelids during a blink is not constant and varies from individual to indivual. The highest velocities obtained half-way the closing of the upper eyelid are from 15 to 30 cm/sec (Doane, 1980; Holly, 1985). The duration of the closing phase is about 80 msec and the duration of the opening phase 175 msec (Doane, 1980).

Periodic blinking is the usual denomination of the involuntary, usually unconscious, quick eye closures that occur throughout the day. In relaxed adults the average frequency of periodic blinking is 15 to 16 per minute, the range being 3 to 28 per minute (Drew,1951). Stimuli may provoke an increase in the blinking frequency, eliciting reflex blinks. The velocity of the eyelid movement is not changed. The reflex blink elicited by a stimulus occurs with a latency of about 100 msec. The reflex blink can also eliminate very quickly the stimulus, such as an instilled ophthalmic drop, from the eye surface. Several stimuli, such as bright light (flash), loud noise, nasal irritation and wearing contact lenses (Hill and Carney, 1984; Carney, 1984) may provoke reflex blinking. If the eye is approached by a foreign body (e.g. the bottle dropper or a light touch to the cornea by foreign matter) reflex blinking may also be elicited (Walsh and Hoyt, 1969b). In the experiments of Sorensen and Jensen (1979), reflex blinking seems to be responsible for the very quick decay of the radioactivity during the two first minutes immediately after the instillation of the suspension containing a radioactive tracer.

PROPERTIES OF THE PREPARATION INFLUENCING THE DRUG RETENTION

1) Instilled volume

When eyedrops are administered, the instilled solution is mixed with the precorneal tear film at the eye surface and with the tears in the conjunctival sac. From the work of Benedetto et al. (1984), it appears that at most 3 µl of additional solution can be mixed with the precorneal tear film. Mishima et al. (1966) demonstrated that the cul de sac cannot hold an additional amount of more than 25 µl unless the solution is added slowly to allow blinking and drainage.

According to Zaki et al. (1986) the instillation of a 30 µl drop into the human eye causes reflex blinking, which splashes a considerable proportion (20% to 30%) of the dose onto the eyelashes. The instillation into humans of 20 µl and 50 µl 0.5% pilocarpine hydrocloride solution gives equivalent miotic responses (File and Patton, 1980). Ludwig and Van Ooteghem (1986a) registered the decay of fluorescence on the eye surface after instillation of 20 µl, and of smaller volumes of solutions containing fluorescein. The decrease of the fluorescence is slower when 1 µl is instilled than when 20 µl drops are used. The difference between the two elimination rates, however, is not significant. To obtain a maximal retention on the eye surface and to reduce the side effects of drugs, the administration of drops with a maximal volume of 20 µl is preferable. The use of special eye droppers delivering drops smaller than 20 µl is also advisable.

2) Osmolality

The osmolality of tears is directly proportional to the number of dissolved ions and crystalloids. Proteins, because of their molecular weight and low concentrations, contribute only slightly to the total osmotic pressure. The tonicity of human tears is influenced by the evaporation process when the eye is open. The osmolality after prolonged eye closure or during sleep is 293 to 288 mOsm/Kg (Terry and Hill, 1978). After the eye is opened, the osmolality varies from 302 to 318 mOsm/Kg (Gilbard and Farris, 1978; Farris et al. 1981; Terry and Hill, 1978; Benjamin and Hill, 1983). During the day, the osmolality progresses at a rate of 1.43 mOsm/Kg.hr (Benjamin and Hill 1983).

An ophthalmic solution instilled in the eye is mixed with the tears present. The osmotic pressure of the mixture then depends upon the osmolality of the tears and of that of the instilled solution. If the osmotic pressure obtained is within definite limits, no discomfort is experienced; beyond these values irritation takes place, eliciting reflex tears and reflex blinking. The osmolalities of the ophthalmic solutions provoking discomfort or irritation have been determined by different authors (Table 1).

Table 1 : Osmolalities of irritant solutions

Osmolality (mOsm/Kg)	Authors
<100	Bisantis et al. (1982)
<266	Riegelmann and Vaughan (1958)
	Trolle Lassen (1958)
>445	Trolle Lassen (1958)
>480	Riegelman and Vaughan (1958)
>640	Maurice (1971)
	Bisantis et al. (1982)
	Ludwig and Van Ooteghem (1986b)

The original osmolality of the tear film is regained 1 to 2 minutes after the instillation of the non-isotonic solution (Holly and Lamberts, 1981). This is mainly due to a rapid flow of water across the cornea (Mishima, 1965). The instillation of a hypotonic drug solution creates an osmotic gradient between the tear film and the surrounding tissues. This induces a flow of water from the eye surface to the cornea, increasing temporarily the drug concentration on the eye surface (Barendsen et al. 1979).

3) pH

The pH of tears is influenced by the dissolved substances, some of which form buffer systems (e.g. bicarbonate - carbon dioxide). The precorneal tear film forms on the eye surface a very thin film with a thickness of about 8 µm. When the eyelids are open the pH of precorneal tear film increases through evaporation of carbon dioxide. When the eyelids remain open for

50 seconds an equilibration with the partial pressure of carbon dioxide of the environment might occur, and the pH would increase to 9.3 (Fisher and Wiederholt, 1982).

The pH of the tears has been determined by several authors. A summary of the values obtained is given by Carney and Hill (1976). The mean value seems to be 7.4, but there are important variations.

After an ophthalmic solution is instilled on the eye surface, it is mixed with the tears present in the conjunctival sac and with the precorneal tear film. The pH of the mixture is mainly determined by the pH of the instilled solution. If the pH of the mixture reaches certain values, reflex tears and reflex blinking are elicited. These values depend, however, on the composition of the instilled solution and on the contact time between the solution and the corneal surface. The influence of the pH of instilled solutions is summarized in Table 2.

Table 2 : The influence of the pH of ophthalmic solutions

Solution		Influence	Authors
Composition	pH		
lake water	4.6	brief congestion	Basu et al. (1982)
10% phenilephrine	4.8	reflex tear	Coles & Jaros (1984)
citrate buffer	5.0	" "	Norn (1985)
isotonic solution	< 5.8	irritation	Trolle-Lassen (1958)
1% tropicamide	5.0	reflex tear	Coles & Jaros (1984)
lake water	6.3	brief congestion	Basu et al. (1982)
citrate buffer	< 6.4	irritation	Bisantis et al. (1982)
borate buffer	> 8.5	"	Bisantis et al. (1982)
borate buffer	9.0	reflex tear	Norn (1985)
isotonic solution	> 9.7	irritation	Trolle-Lassen (1958)

The irritant solution is neutralized by reflex tears and drainage. Since the tears have a very limited buffer capacity and only the superficial layer of the tear film is eliminated by the movement of the eyelids, the neutralization takes at least several minutes (Norn, 1985).

4) Viscosity

The viscosity of ophthalmic solutions is often increased in order to obtain a prolonged retention of drugs on the eye surface. The irritation and the reflex tearing caused by the instillation of viscous solutions must be examined.

The viscosity of tears is influenced by proteins dissolved in the lacrimal fluid. The viscosity of tears has seldom been determined because it is difficult to collect enough tears for a determination. Hamano and Mitsunaga (1973) recorded with a cone-plate viscosimeter the rheograms of rabbit tears. The viscosity depended upon the rate of shear, indicating a non-Newtonian behavior. These tears had also a yield value of about 0.03 Pa.s.

Schuller et al. (1972) have determined the correlation between the viscosities of human tears, measured with a capillary viscosimeter, and the complaints of patients wearing contact lenses. The viscosity of human tears ranges from 1.3 to 5.9 mPa.s with a mean value of 2.916 mPa.s. Patients with tears viscosities higher than 2.5 mPa.s are too prone to symptoms of burning, dryness and general discomfort to wear contact lenses.

During the closing of the eyelids the tear film on the eye surface is submitted to a shear movement. The precorneal tear film has a thickness of about 8 µm; the mean velocity of the upper eyelid movement during the closure is about 16 cm/sec. Therefore the rate would also be 20,000 sec . On the other hand tha lid force needed to move the upper eyelid downward would vary from 0.2 N to 0.8 N and the pain threshold would be 0.9 N (Hung et al. 1977). Consequently the viscosity of the tears would vary from 65.4 to 261.6 mPa.s. A painful sensation would be observed at a viscosity of 297.6 mPa.s. These calculated viscosity values seem to be very high, perhaps due to a lack of precision in the determination of the forces needed to close the eyelids.

5) Drugs and adjuvants

Drugs and adjuvants, which may influence tear secretion and blink frquency, can also influence the retention of a drug at the eye surface and the bioavailability. Drugs administered systemically or applied topically might also have an influence.

In Table 3 the influence of systemic drugs is summarized.

Table 3 : Influence of drugs administered sistemically (Grandall and Leopold, 1979)

STIMULATION OF TEAR FLOW

- Muscarinic drugs (e.g. pilocarpine, carbochol, neostigmine...)
- Sympathomimetics (epinephrine, ephedrine...)
- Antihypertensives (reserpine, diazoxide)
- Antimetabolite (fluorouracil)
- Miscellaneous (chronic heroin use, histamine...)

REDUCTION OF TEAR FLOW

- Antimuscarinic drugs (atropine, scopolamine)
- Antihistamines
- Beta-adrenergic blocker (practolol)
- General anesthetics (nitrous oxide, halothae, enflurane)
- Miscellaneous (phenazopyridine HCl)

Generally, only the influence of the tear secretion has been studied, but in some cases drugs influence both the tear secretion and the blink frequency. General anaesthetics may completely inhibit the lid movements (Dundee et al., 1982). When prescribing ophthalmic solutions it is very important to know which other drugs are used by the patients.

In Table 4 the influence of some drugs applied topically and of some adjuvants are summarized.

Table 4 - Influence of drugs applied topically and of adjuvants (Burstein 1985; Norn & Opauszki 1977)

DRUGS:	Timolol	reduces tear flow
	Topical anesthetics	reduce tear flow
	Topical anesthetics	reduce blinking frequency
	Metipranolol	stimulates tear flow
	Pilocarpine	stimulates tear flow
	Antazoline HCl	stimulates tear flow
ADJUVANTS:	Benzalkonium chloride	disrupts tear film
	Chlorhexidine digluc.	no effect
	Thiomersal	no effect
	Phenilmercuric nitr.	no effect
	Methylcellulose	increases stability of tear film
	PVA	increases stability of tear film
	Dextran	no effect

The influence of antazoline on the tear flow of ten volunteers has been studied. Solutions of 1.0 or 1.5% antazoline and sodium chloride solutions with the same osmolality were used. Different volumes of the solutions were first instilled, then solutions with different osmolarities. The influence of the drug was measured by determining the overflow onto the cheek: the overflow was absorbed on a cotton tip within 60 seconds of administration. The overflow values, determined by the weight increase of the cotton-wool tip, are indicated in Table 5.

Table 5 - Influence of antazoline HCl on the overflow (µl)

1. Influence of the instillation of isotonic solution

instilled volume	0.90% NaCl	1.50% antazoline HCl 0.62% NaCl
10 µl	3 µl	---
30 µl	9 µl	98 µl
50 µl	30 µl	136 µl

2. Influence of the osmolality (instilled volume, 50 µl)

Osmolality (mOsm/Kg)	NaCl	1% antazoline HCl + NaCl	1.50% antazoline HCl + NaCl
61	32 µl	105 µl	---
285	30 µl	102 µl	136 µl
589	34 µl	---	---

The overflow of the normal saline indicates that only a part of the instilled 50 µl remains on the eye surface. Only 20 µl can be added to the present tear film. Nor is the overflow influenced by osmolalities lower than 589 mOsm/Kg or a 1.8% NaCl solution. The solutions of antazoline HCl irritate and elicit immediately an important reflex tearing. The reflex tearing cannot be reduced by administering small volumes or isotonic solutions.

The most important factor influencing the retention of a drug seems to be the properties of the drug itself. If the drug irritates the eye, it appears extremely difficult to obtain a long retention at the eye surface.

CONCLUSION

The retention of a drug on the eye surface is determined by the amount of tear flow and by the blinking frequency. These can be stimulated by different factors. The most important factors, however, are the properties of the administered drugs. If the drug is not an irritant, it is possible to increase the retention time by instillation of small drops, by adjusting the osmolality and the pH, and by choosing the appropiate adjuvants.

REFERENCES

Barendsen H., Oosterhuis J.A., Van Haeringen N.J. (1979). Concentration of fluoresceine in tear fluid after instillation as eyedrops: II Hypotonic eyedrops. Ophthalmic Res. 11: 83-89.

Basu P.K., Avaria M., Hasany S.M. (1982). Effect of acidic lake water on the eye. Can. J. Ophthalmol. 17: 74-78.

Benedetto D.A. (1982). In vivo observation of tear dynamics. Invest. Ophthalmol. Vis. Sci. 21 (ARVO suppl.): 221.

Benedetto D.A., Cinch T.E., Laibson P.R. (1984). In vivo observations of tear dynamics using fluorophotometry. Arch. Ophthalmol. 102: 410-412.

Benjamin W.J, Hill R.M. (1983). Human tears: osmotic characteristics. Invest. Ophthalmol. Vis. Sci. 24: 1624-1626.

Bisantis C., Squeri C.A., Colsi P., Provenzano P., Trombetta C. (1982). Sur l'usage des collyres hypo-,iso- et hyper-osmotiques, acides ou alcalins, dans le diagnostic et le traitment des anomalies de la secretion des larmes. Bull. Memoir. Soc. Fran. Ophthalmol. 94 : 75-78.

Burstein N.L. (1985). The effects of topical drugs and preservatives on the tears and corneal epithelium in dry eye. Trans. Ophthalmol. Soc. UK 104: 402-409.

Carney L.G., Hill R.M. (1976). Human tear pH: diurnal variations. Arch. Ophthalmol. 94: 821-824.

Carney L.G. (1984). Variation in blinking behaviour during soft lens wear. Int. Contact Lens Clin. 11: 249-252.

Coles W.H., Jaros P.A. (1984). Dynamics of ocular surface pH. Br. J. Ophthalmol. 68: 549-552.

Doane M.G. (1979). Dynamics of the human eyeblink. Invest. Ophthalmol. Vis. Sci. 18 (ARVO suppl.):198.

Doane M.G. (1980). Interaction of eyelids and tears in corneal wetting and the dynamics of the normal human eyeblink. Am. J. Ophthalmol. 89: 507-516.

Drew G.C. (1951). Variations in reflex blink-rate during visual-motor tasks. Quart. J. Exp. Psychol. 3: 73-88.

Dundee J.M., Hassard T.H., McGovan W.A., Henshaw J. (1982). The "induction" dose of thiopentone. A method of study and preliminary illustrative results. Anaesthesia 37: 1176-1184.

Farris R.L., Stuchell R.N., Mandel I.D. (1981). Basal and reflex human tear analysis. I Physical measurements: osmolarity, basal volumes and reflex flow rate. Ophthalmology (Rochester) 88:852-57.

File R.R., Patton T.F. (1980). Topically applied pilocarpine. Arch. Ophthalmol. 98: 112-115.

Fisher F.H., Weiderholt M. (1982). Human precorneal tear film pH measured by microelectrodes. Graefes Arch. Clin. Exp. Opthalmol 218:168-170.

Gilbard P.J., Farris R.L. (1978). Osmolarity of tear microvolumes in keratoconjunctivitis sicca. Arch. Ophthalmol. 96: 677-681.

Grandall D.C., Leopold D.H. (1979). The influence of systemic drugs on tear constituents. Ophthalmogy (Rochester) 86: 115-125.

Hamano H., Mitsunaga S. (1973). Viscosity of rabbit tears. Jap. J. Ophthalmol. 17: 290-299.

Hawes M.J., Ellis P.P. (1985). Tearing in geriatic patient: causes and treatments. Geriatrics 38: 113-121.

Hill R.M., Carney L.G. (1984). The effects of hard lens wear on blinking behavior. Int. Ophthalmol. Clin. 14: 242-248.

Holly F.J., Lamberts D.W. (1981). Effect of non isotonic solutions on tear film osmolality. Invest. Ophthalmol. Vis. Sci. 20: 236-245.

Holly F.J. (1985). Ocular wetting: basic concepts, measurememnts and applicability: hydrodynamics of blinking and contact lens wear. Frontiers in lacrymology, Seminar Series, Dry Eye Institute, Lubbock TX 79499 p 60.

Hung G., Hsu F., Stark L. (1977). Dynamics of the human eye blink. Am. J. Optom. Physiol. Opt. 54: 678-690.

Jordan A.J., Baum J.L. (1979). On the nature of physiologic flow. Invest. Ophthalmol. Vis. Sci. 18 (ARVO suppl.): 197.

Jordan A.J., Baum J.L. (1980). Basic tear flow - does it exist? Ophthalmology (Rochester) 87: 920-930.

Lamberts D.W., Foster C.S., Perry H.D. (1979). Schirmer test after topical anaesthesia and the tear meniscus height in normal eyes. Arch. Ophthalmol. 97: 1082-1085.

Ludwig A., Van Ooteghem M. (1986a). The influence of the drop size on the elimination of an ophthalmic solution from the precorneal area of human eyes. Drug Develop. Ind. Pharm. 12: 2231-2242.

Ludwig A., Van Ooteghem M. (1986b). The influence of the osmolality on the precorneal retention of ophthalmic solutions. J. Pharm. Belg., in press.

Maurice D.M. (1971). The tonicity of an eye drop and its dilution by tears. Exp. Eye Res. 11: 30-33.

Mishima S. (1965). Some physiological aspects of the precorneal tear film. Arch. Ophthalmol. 73: 233-241.

Mishima S., Gasset A., Klyce S.O., Baum J.L. (1966). Determination of tear volume and tear flow. Invest. Ophthalmol. Vis. Sci. 5: 264-266.

Norn M.S., Opauszki A. (1977). Effects of ophthalmic vehicles on the stability of the precorneal film. Acta Ophthalmol. (Copenh.) 55: 23-24.

Norn M. (1985). Tear pH after instillation of buffer in vivo. Acta Ophthalmol. (Copenh.) 63 (suppl. 173): 32-34.

Riegelman S., Vaughan D.G. (1958). Ophthalmic solutions. J. Am. Pharm. Ass., Pract. Ed. 8: 474-477.

Rolando M., Refojo M.F. (1983). Tear evaporimeter for measuring water evaporation rate from the tear film under controlled conditions in humans. Exp. Eye Res. 36: 25-83.

Schuller W.O., Yang W.H., Hill R.M. (1972). Clinical measurements of tears. J. Am. Optom. Ass. 43: 1358-1361.

Sorensen B., Jensen F.T. (1979). Tear flow in normal human eyes. Determination by means of radioisotope and gamma camera. Acta Ophthalmol. (Copenh.) 57: 564-581.

Terry J.E., Hill R.M. (1978). Human tear osmotic pressure, diurnal variations and the closed eye. Arch. Ophthalmol. 96: 120-122.

Trolle-Lassen C. (1958). Investigations in to the sensitivity of the human eye to hypo- and hypertonic solutions as well as solutions with unphysiological hydrogen ion concentrations. Pharm. Weekbl. 93: 148-155.

Walsh F.B., Hoyt W.F. (1969a). Clinical neuroophthalmology, Williams & Wilkins, Baltimore pp. 551-555.

Walsh F.B., Hoyt W.F. (1969b). Clinical neuroophthalmology, Williams & Wilkins, Baltimore pp. 318-328.

Wright P. (1985). Normal tear production and drainage. Trans. Ophthalmol. Soc. UK 104: 351-354.

Zaki I., Fitzgerald P., Hardy J.G., Wilson C.G. (1986). A comparison of the effect of viscosity on the precorneal residence of solutions in rabbit and man. J. Pharm. Pharmacol. 38: 463-466.

KINETICS OF TOPICALLY APPLIED OPHTHALMIC DRUGS

D.M. Maurice

Division of Ophthalmology
Stanford University, Stanford, California, USA

The more important aspects of the behavior of drugs in the tear film and after penetration into the eye are described. The kinetics of lipophilic molecules is differentiated from that of hydrophilic. The importance of the lens as a reservoir is suggested.

INTRODUCTION

The behavior of a drug applied as a drop to the eye may be divided into two phases: that which occurs while it is in the tear film and that after its penetration into the ocular tissues. This review will consider each phase in turn, and will distinguish between drugs which are hydrophilic, whose kinetics can be accounted for by two-compartment theory, and those which are lipophilic, whose behavior is still little understood.

TEAR KINETICS

A drop dispensed from a standard bottle tip has a volume of about 40 µl, but only a fraction of this is retained between the eyelids, the amount depending on how much the patient squeezes in response to its arrival. The increased volume resulting from the instillation drains out rapidly largely in consequence of blinks, each one of which will remove about 2 µl of excess tear fluid (Maurice, 1973). During this time the fluid in the interpalpebral space, which at first must be close in concentration to the drop, begins to mix with the tear fluid under the lids, as illustrated in Fig. 1. The concentration of drug in the tear fluid that would result from complete mixing is found to be only about a quarter of that in the drop.

After the initial mixing, the drug is gradually flushed out of the conjunctival sac by the flow of freshly secreted tears. This flow rate can be very much increased by eye drops that sting, but it is not affected by the frequency of blinking nor by anesthesia. In normal people the washout rate will reduce the concentration of a drug in the tear film to one-tenth of its starting value in about 20 min, but this figure shows considerable variation and is often much quicker. The rate of loss in the rabbit eye is similar, but because the animal blinks infrequently, the concentration profile tends to conform to a series of diminishing plateaux rather than a smooth exponential fall.

For the hydrophilic drugs this is the principal way in which a drug is lost from the conjunctival sac. On the other hand, it seems that many lipophilic drugs leave the tear film more rapidly because they can penetrate into the conjunctival and corneal epithelium faster than they are lost by drainage. The rate of loss of pilocarpine from the conjunctival sac of the rabbit is such that it drops to one-tenth in about 4 min (Sieg and Robinson, 1976; Urtti and

Ophthalmic Drug Delivery. Biopharmaceutical, Technological and Clinical Aspects.
M.S. Saettone, G. Bucci, P. Speiser (eds.) Fidia Research Series, vol. 11, Liviana Press, Padova © 1987

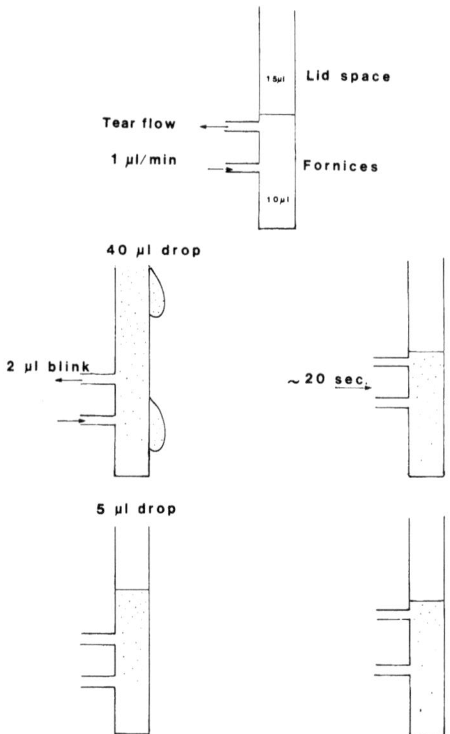

Figure 1.
Schematic representation of relationship of conjunctival tear fluid and an instilled drop of large and small volume showing penetration of drug into fornices.

The lower part of the contained volume represents the tear fluid normally present in the eye; the upper part, the excess fluid held between the lid margins.

Salminen, 1986). It can be expected that after drainage has sufficiently lowered the concentration in the tear film, a small fraction of the drug will pass back into the fluid from the conjunctival cells. This can give rise to a slowing down in the rate of drop in tear film concentration. Prolonged entry of drug into the tears may also take place from depots on the lid margins, especially if ointments are used.

It may be noted at this point that the movement of water by osmotic forces across the conjunctival surface is very rapid because of its large area and the thinness of the tear layer. In consequence, a hypertonic solution will be diluted to isotonicity in a few seconds. An increased exposure of the cornea to a drug will not follow its instillation at a concentration so high as to make the drop hypertonic but rather may lead only to a greater systemic absorption.

Some drugs may cause unpleasant systemic side effects as a result of their absorption across the conjunctiva and nasolacrimal duct. For a given systemic effect, which will correspond to the instillation of a fixed mass of drug between the lids, the initial tear film concentration should be greater if the drop volume in which this mass is dissolved is small, because then less will be lost by rapid drainage; accordingly, the therapeutic index should be larger when microdrops are used. Of course, the drug dissolved in the portion of the drop that runs down the cheeks does not affect the index because it neither penetrates the eye nor the skin.

CORNEAL PENETRATION

The penetration into the eye of most drugs, except the very lipophilic ones, is controlled by the corneal epithelium. From a practical point of view the penetration can be expressed as the maximum concentration of the drug achieved in the aqueous humor divided by its concentration in the drop (Fig. 2). Some published data for the human eye are collected in Table 1. Lipid soluble chloramphenicol penetrates 100 times more readily than the hydrophilic gentamicin.

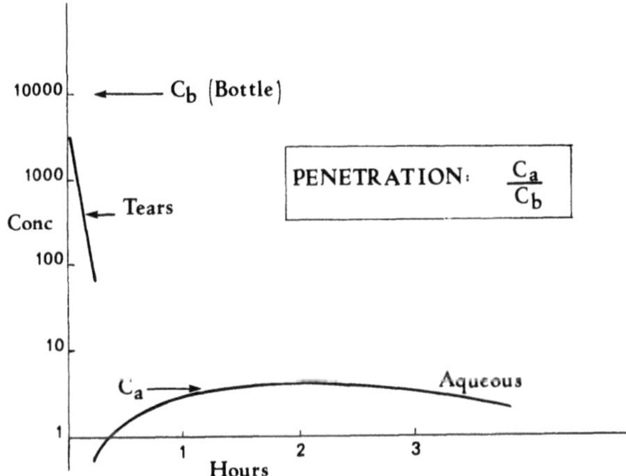

Figure 2
A functional definition of drug penetration relating the maximum concentration in the anterior chamber to that in the instilled drop.

Fluorescein does not stain the epithelium during its passage. On the other hand, the lipid-soluble fluorescent dye rhodamine B can be seen in the slit lamp to stain the cell layer heavily in the early stages after its administration, though later its concentration becomes more uniform across the cornea (Guss, Johnson and Maurice, 1984). Similar behavior is exhibited by the lipophilic therapeutic drugs hydrocortisone and pilocarpine.

The corneal stroma acts as a depot to a hydrophilic drug after it has penetrated the epithelium, and then it is slowly transferred into the aqueous humor across the endothelium, which controls its rate of passage. The kinetics of such drugs in the anterior chamber are well represented over two decades of concentration by a double exponential equation.

TABLE I

Functional penetration of various drugs after a single drop instillation in the human eye

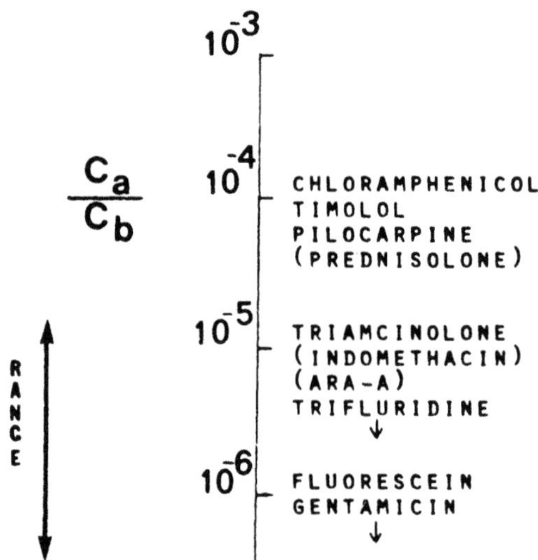

The figures are only approximate, and the range of values for the more poorly penetrating ones is shown on the left. The drugs in parentheses were applied in suspension. The levels of trifluridine and gentamicin represent the upper limits of sensitivity. The references will be found in the bibliography.

On the other hand, the changes of anterior chamber concentration with time for the lipophilic drugs do not seem to fit any simple multiexponential relationship (Fig. 3). The explanation of the shape of the curve may have to take into consideration at least the following factors:

1) Concentration dependence of permeability and diffusion constants
2) Binding to the tissues
3) Diffusion into unstirred tissue volumes
4) Division of the cornea into separate epithelial and stromal compartments

INFLUENCE OF LENS

A clue to the behavior of lipophilic drugs in the anterior chamber may be found in that of the hydrophilic fluorescein at long times after its application to the eye. After the anterior chamber concentration has undergone its two decades of exponential drop, its rate of fall diminishes sharply and the corneal level becomes close to that of the aqueous. This can be attributed to a diffusion back into the aqueous humor of the dye that penetrated into the lens in the early stages (Fig. 4). The diffusion of the lipophilic rhodamine B into the lens is much more notable than that of fluorescein, and only 1 hr after its instillation into the eye of a rabbit, the outer lens cortex is the most brilliantly stained tissue visible by the slit lamp.

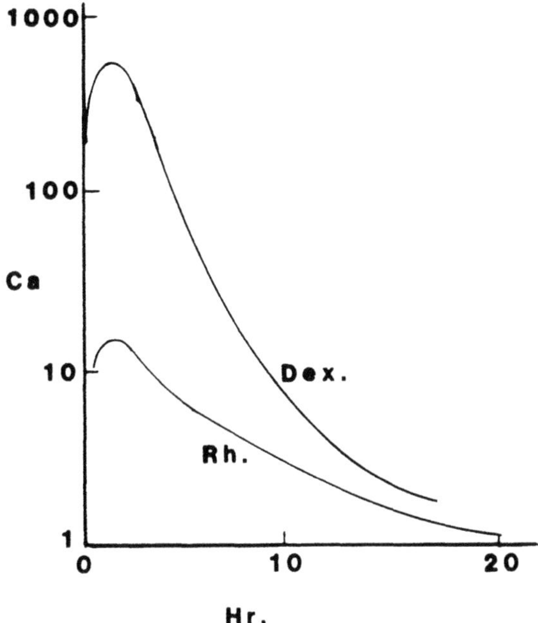

Figure 3.
Changes of aqueous humor concentration (arbitrary units) with time after the instillation of drops of dexamethasone and rhodamine B.

Without calling the listed factors 1, 2 and 4 into play, I suggest that after a period of about 30 minutes, the aqueous humor concentration of rhodamine starts on a simple exponential drop, which is slowed after about 2 hours by the return of the dye from the lens and possibly in part from the iris or ciliary body. This hypothesis could be tested by the application of heat diffusion theory, which has been able to account for the behavior of fluorescein in the lens (Kaiser and Maurice, 1964). Unfortunately, the lateral diffusion of the drug beyond the margins of the pupil will seriously complicate the computation for longer periods of time.

Appreciable concentrations of therapeutic drugs, for example, dexamethasone (Hamard et al., 1975), pilocarpine (Makoid and Robinson, 1979) and flurbiprofen (Anderson and Chen, 1982) are found in the lens after their instillation into the rabbit eye. The concentrations were determined for the lens as a whole, and very much higher levels must be expected in the outer cortex, which is where the drug must be located. If the suggested mechanism is correct, the repeated instillations of a drug over a long period of time could result in a heavy loading of the lens, and this could lead to a significant return to the anterior chamber and a leveling out of the troughs in concentration that are to be expected between drops, especially during sleep. Additionally, after a delay period, lateral diffusion could lead to drug delivery to the posterior segment of the eye via the lens cortex.

PROLONGED RELEASE

Many attempts have been made to prolong the action of a drug in the eye by delaying its release into the tears. A distinction needs to be made between pulse delivery and true prolonged delivery. The latter occurs when the rate of loss of drug from the tears is slower than the loss from the eye in consequence of its natural intraocular kinetics--usually, the time constant imposed by the combination of the stromal depot and the endothelial barrier of the cornea (Fig. 5). Pulse delivery, on the other hand, corresponds to the rate of tear film loss being faster than that from the eye. It results in a high initial penetration of drug in the eye that insures an extension of its action but at the risk of greater ocular and systemic toxicity. Often the extended action of a drug like pilocarpine resulting from pulsed delivery is mistaken for prolonged delivery, because the saturation of its biological effect conceals that a very high concentration has been created in the anterior chamber.

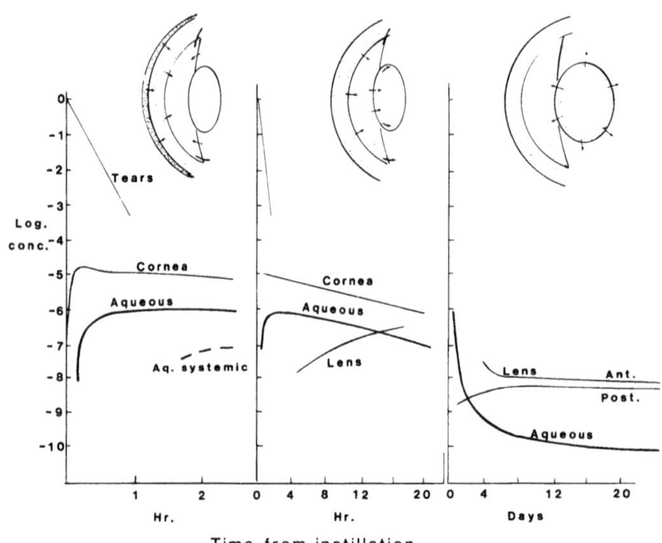

Figure 4

The relative concentration in the tissues and fluids of the eye after the instillation of a single drop of fluorescein. Three phases are illustrated: 1) penetration from the tears 2) fall in concentration controlled by the corneal endothelium; human data is available for these phases, and the rabbit data is similar 3) fall in concentration controlled by return of dye from the lens; only rabbit data is available.

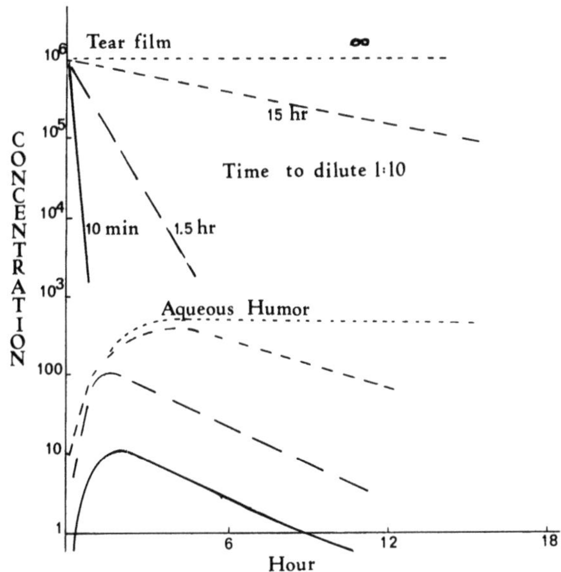

Figure 5
The distinction between pulse and prolonged delivery

The upper part shows various rates of concentration decline in the tear film; the lower part shows the corresponding concentration profiles in the aqueous humor, where the natural loss coefficient leads to a 10 times fall in concentration in 6 hr.

The drug tear concentration normally drops 10 times in 10 minutes. If this is artificially slowed, ninefold, to 1 1/2 hr, the rate of decline is still faster than the natural loss coefficient of the aqueous humor; the aqueous profile is not changed but only raised in magnitude by a factor of nine; this is pulse delivery. If the rate of loss from the tear film is slowed tenfold more, this becomes slower than the natural loss from the aqueous humor, and its profile is extended; this is prolonged delivery.

This work was supported by National Institutes of Health Grant EY 00431.

REFERENCES

Adler CA, Maurice DM, Paterson ME (1971) The effect of viscosity of the vehicle on the penetration of fluorescein into the human eye. Exp Eye Res 11:34-42.
Anderson JA, Chen CC, Vita JB, Shackleton M (1982) Disposition of topical flurbiprofen in normal and aphakic rabbit eyes. Arch Ophthalmol 100:642-645.
Beasley H, Boltralik JJ, Baldwin HA (1975) Chloramphenicol in aqueous humor after topical application. Arch Ophthalmol 93:184-185.
Ellerhorst B, Golden B, Nabil J (1975) Ocular penetration of topically applied gentamicin. Arch Ophthalmol 93:371-379.
Guss R, Johnson F, Maurice D (1984) Rhodamine B as a test molecule in intraocular dynamics. Invest Ophthalmol Vis Sci 25:758-762.
Hamard H, Schmitt C, Plazonnet B, LeDouarec JS (1975) Étude de la penetration oculaire de la dexamethasone. In: DeMailly P, Hamard H, Luton JP (eds): Oeil et cortisone. Masson and Cie, Paris; pp. 3-81.
Kaiser RJ, Maurice DM (1964) The diffusion of fluorescein in the lens. Exp Eye Res 3:156-165.
Krohn DL (1978) Flux of topical pilocarpine to the human aqueous. Trans Am Soc Ophthalmol 76:502-527.
Leibowitz HM, Berrospi AR, Kupferman A, Restropo GV, Galvis V, Alvarez JA (1977) Penetration of topically administered prednisolone acetate into the human aqueous humor. Am J Ophthalmol 83:402-406.
Makoid MC, Robinson JR (1979) Pharmacokinetics of topically applied pilocarpine in the albino rabbit eye. J Pharm Sci 68:435-443.
Maurice DM, Mishima S (1984) Ocular pharmacokinetics. In: Sears ML Handbook of experimental pharmacokinetics. Springer Verlag, Berlin; pp. 19-116.
Maurice DM (1973) The dynamics and drainage of tears. Intl Ophthalmol Clin 13:103-116.
Pavan-Langston D, Nelson DJ (1979) Intraocular penetration of trifluridine. Am J Ophthalmol 87:814-818.
Phillips CI, Bartholomew RS, Ghulamqadir K, Schmitt CJ, Vogen R (1981) Penetration of timolol eye drops into human aqueous humour. Br J Ophthalmol 65:593-595.
Poirier RH, Kinkel AW, Ellison AC, Lewis R (1975) Intraocular penetration of topical 3% adenine arabinoside. In: Pavan-Langston D, Buchanan RA, Alford, CA (eds): Adenine arabinoside: an antiviral agent. Raven Press, New York: pp. 307-312.
Sanders DR, Goldstick B, Kraff C, Hutchins R, Bernstein MS, Evasn MA (1983) Aqueous penetration of oral and topical indomethacin in humans. Arch Ophthalmol 101:1614-1616.
Sieg JW, Robinson JR (1976) Mechanistic studies on transcorneal permeation of pilocarpine. J Pharm Sci 65:1816-1822.
Sugar J, Burde RM, Sugar A, Waltman SR, Kripalani KJ, Weliky I, Becker B (1972) Tetrahydrotriamcinolone and triamcinolone I. Ocular penetration. Invest Ophthalmol 11:890-893.
Urtti A, Salminen, L (1986) Concentration-dependent precorneal loss of pilocarpine in rabbit eyes. Acta Ophthalmol (in press).

Where no citations are provided in support of statements in this text, they will be found in the chapter by Maurice and Mishima (1984).

LATICES AND THERMOSENSITIVE GELS AS SUSTAINED DELIVERY SYSTEMS TO THE EYE

R. Gurny, H. Ibrahim, T. Boye and P. Buri

School of Pharmacy, University of Geneva
30, Quai Ernest-Ansermet, CH-1211 Geneva 4, Switzerland

Traditionally, ophthalmic formulations have been limited to solutions or ointments and in some rare cases to emulsions or suspensions. An alternative is the use of carefully selected pH-sensitive polymeric materials dispersed in water in the nanometer size range as carriers or polymers with interesting sol-gel transition behavior. These two systems have been formulated and further investigated in order to slow down the extremely rapid drug exchange between the tear fluid and the medicament.

INTRODUCTION

In recent years, several colloidal preparations for ophthalmic use have been investigated, based on nanoparticles or liposomes. However, little evidence could be found in most cases of considerable advantage over conventional formulations. In contrast, the introduction in the early eighties of the concept of *in situ* gel formation by means of highly concentrated latex systems demonstrated that a considerable prolongation in duration of action could be obtained (Gurny and Taylor (1980)). This had previously been achieved only with inserts. In the past 15 years, the coating technology developed in the paint industry has been the driving force for the very rapid evolution in the field of aqueous dispersions of polymers. Polymers with solubility properties depending on the pH, such as cellulose derivatives, cannot be prepared by emulsion polymerization techniques. An alternative method for the preparation of polymeric dispersions in the nanometer size range is the emulsification of the polymers, their solutions or melts into water, using conventional emulsifiers, stabilizer and emulsification techniques. Different approaches for the preparation of these so-called "latex formulations" are possible, e.g., solution emulsification, phase inversion, self-emulsification (Vanderhoff, El- Aasser and Ungelstad (1979)). Recent advances in our knowledge of *in situ* gel forming systems used via the ocular route by drug-carrying systems have been made. The systems are based on the mechanism of drug adsorption onto the surface of colloidal particles (0.3 µm average particle size) which show good biocompatibility.

Another *in situ* gel formation by thermogelation for the occular route was first mentioned by Miller and Donovan (1982) using thermosetting gels obtained from the poloxamers. A general attempt to classify therapeutic systems is made by Heilman (1978) were a distinction is made between diffusion units, osmotic units and soluble units. A further classification for the soluble units is given in Table 1:

Ophthalmic Drug Delivery. Biopharmaceutical, Technological and Clinical Aspects.
M.S. Saettone, G. Bucci, P. Speiser (eds.) Fidia Research Series, vol. 11, Liviana Press, Padova

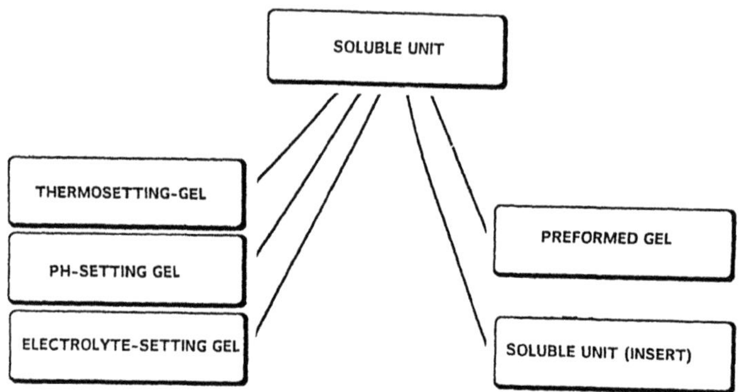

Figure 1
Classification of Soluble Therapeutic Units
for Sustained Drug Delivery to the Eye

In this investigation only the thermosetting and pH-setting gels will be mentioned. The idealized behavior of such ophthalmic systems is given in Figure 2, where in both cases an increase in viscosity is expected due to a temperature or pH effect.

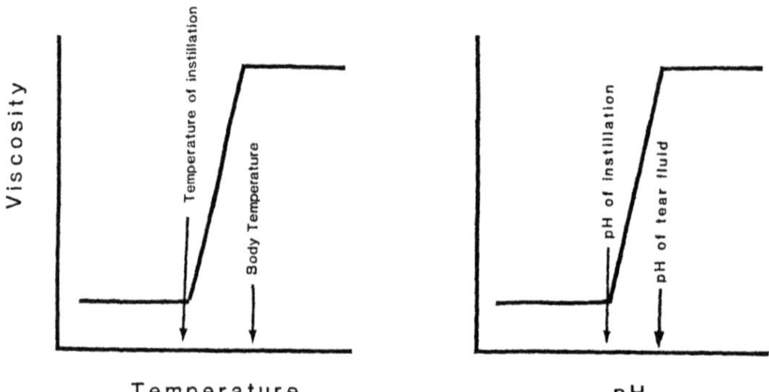

Figure 2
Idealized Viscosity Behavior of *in situ*
Gel Forming Therapeutic Systems

THERMOSETTING-GELS

The particular sol-gel behavior of poloxamers for so-called temperature-sensitive polymeric gels has been investigated. This specific block polymer was chosen since it shows a reversible thermal gelation phenomenon due to the very marked temperature dependence of the micellar size above a certain threshold temperature of about 25°C.

$$HO{-}(CH_2{-}CH_2{-}O)_n{-}(\underset{\displaystyle CH_2}{\underset{|}{CH}}{-}CH_2{-}O)_m{-}(CH_2{-}CH_2{-}O)_n{-}H$$

Figure 3
General Structure of Poloxamer

The hydrophobic/hydrophilic ratio of block polymers can be varied over a large range as well as total molecular weight, typically between 2,000 and 20,000.

It is therefore possible to vary the viscosity as shown in Figure 4.

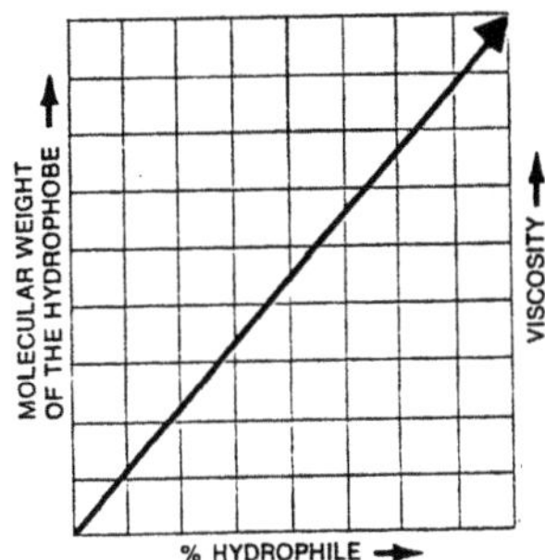

Figure 4
Viscosity of Poloxamers in
Function of their Composition (BASF (1980))

With the increase in hydrophilicity, we get in general a significant decrease in toxicity as shown in Figure 5.

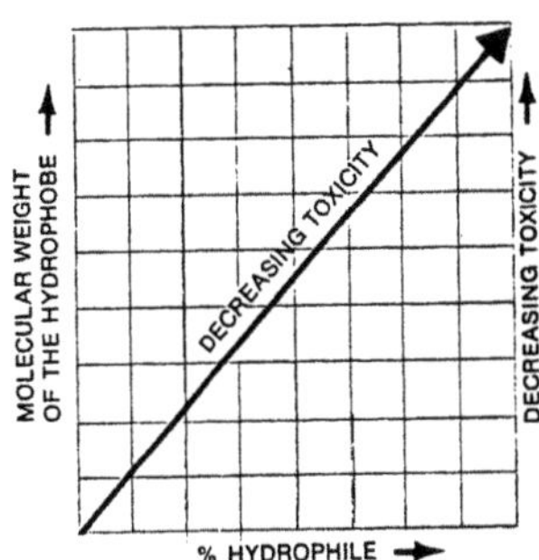

Figure 5
Hydrophilicity as a Function of Toxicity (BASF (1980))

The enthalpy of gelation can be calculated according to Vadnere et al. (1984) by the following equation:

$$\ln c = \frac{\Delta H^{o}_{gel}}{RT_{gel \rightarrow sol}} + \text{constant}$$

where c is the concentration of the polymer in solution, ΔH^{o}_{gel} the enthalpy of transition, and T the temperature.

Several values of enthalpy for various poloxamers are listed in Table 1. It can be seen that there is no linear relation between average molecular weight and the enthalpy of gelation and therefore no criterion for the choice of a suitable polymer. In the present study, the poloxamer 407 was chosen because of it has a low toxicity and gelation enthalpy at low concentrations. It also appears to be an apparent anomaly for poloxamers since the formation of a gel, which is a three-dimensional network more rigid than solution and infinite in extent, would be expected to require a negative entropy change in order to produce a ordered system. If however a ΔH^{o} value is positive, the entropy change will be positive according Eldrige and Ferry (1954).

Poloxamer	Mol.wt.	ΔH^{o}(gel)
F108	14,000	8.0
F 98	13,000	8.1
F127	12,500	9.5
F 88	10,000	6.8
F 68	8,350	5.4
P105	6,500	8.6
P 85	4,600	6.5
P 84	4,200	6.2

Table 1
Enthalpy of Gelation According to Vadnere et al. (1984)

The general investigation of the use of poloxamers as therapeutic systems was attempted with a poloxamer gel, 407 (Pluronic F 127, BASF) at a concentration of 25% wt/wt, using. 4% wt/wt of pilocarpine hydrochloride as an active for glaucoma treatment.

pH-SETTING GELS

The concept of producing a gel *in situ* (e.g. in the conjunctival sac of the eye) from a nanoparticulate system has been developed over the past 7 years (Gurny and Taylor (1980)). The general method for the preparation of pilocarpine-containing nanoparticles by a solvent-removal method is shown schematically in Figure 6 and was described earlier (Gurny et al. (1983)). This method involves the emulsification of an organic solvent solution of the polymer with an aqueous solution of the surfactant, followed by removal of the organic solvent and a fraction of the water. The bioactive material is then added to the dispersion where it is partially adsorbed onto the polymer. It has to be noted that the active material can also be introduced at the beginning in one or the other phase before emulsification. The gel-forming polymers have to be carefully selected in respect to their physico-chemical properties and biocompatibility. Some possible gel-forming polymers for these dispersed systems are given in Table 2.

Chemical structure	Name	Manufacturer	$\bar{M}_w$	A.I.	pK	Observations
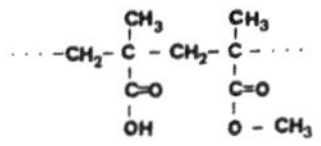 $\cdots -CH_2-C(CH_3)(C{=}O\,OH)-CH_2-C(CH_3)(C{=}O\,O-CH_3)-\cdots$	7203/69A	Röhm Pharma	135000	307	6.1	Monomer ratio 1 : 1
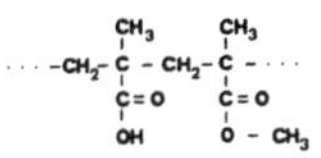 $\cdots -CH_2-C(CH_3)(C{=}O\,OH)-CH_2-C(CH_3)(C{=}O\,O-CH_3)-\cdots$	7203/69B	Röhm Pharma	135000	193	7.1	Monomer ratio 1 : 2
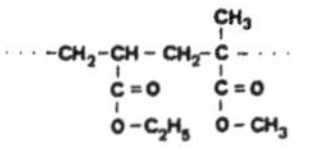 $\cdots -CH_2-CH(C{=}O\,O-C_2H_5)-CH_2-C(CH_3)(C{=}O\,O-CH_3)-\cdots$	7203/58	Röhm Pharma	800000	---	---	Monomer ratio 1 : 1
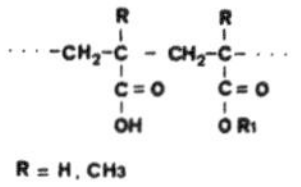 $\cdots -CH_2-C(R)(C{=}O\,OH)-CH_2-C(R)(C{=}O\,OR_1)-\cdots$ R = H, CH_3 R_1 = CH_3, C_2H_5	Eudragit L 30 D	Röhm Pharma	250000	318	6.0	Monomer ratio 1 : 1
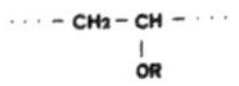 $\cdots -CH_2-CH(OR)-\cdots$ R = H, $COCH_3$, $C_8H_5O_3$	PVAP	Colorcon	25000-40000	205	5.0	Carboxybenzoyl 55 - 65% Acetyl 1.6 - 6.0%
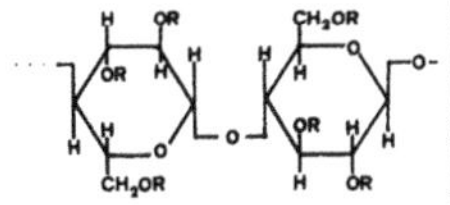 Cellulose chain: H, OR, CH_2OR, OR, H, H, H, O, OR, H, H, CH_2OR, H, OR R = H, CH_3, C_3H_7O, $C_8H_5O_3$, $C_{11}H_{13}O_4$	HPMCP HP-55 "F"	Shin-Etsu	20000	126	5.0	Methoxyl 18.0 - 11.0% Hydroxypropyl 4.0 - 9.0% Carboxybenzoyl 27.0 - 35.0%
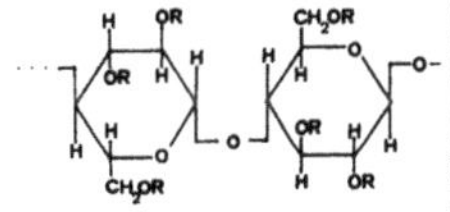 Cellulose chain: H, OR, CH_2OR, OR, H, H, H, O, OR, H, H, CH_2OR, H, OR R = H, $COCH_3$, $C_8H_5O_3$	CAP	Eastman	40000	104	4.9	Combined phthalyl 30.0% - 36.0% Combined acetyl 19.0% - 23.5% Free acid 6% maximum

Table 2
Physico-Chemical Properties of Some Polymers

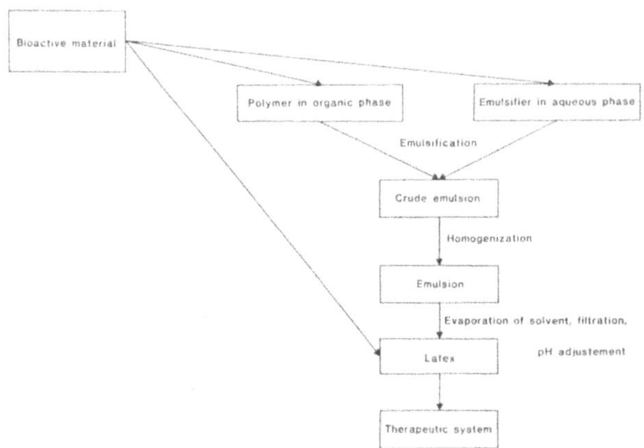

Figure 6
Preparation Scheme of a Polymeric Dispersion

Solubility profiles in water of some selected polymers are shown in Figure 7 and explain very clearly the potential of these macromolecules. However, Figure 8 shows why only cellulose acetate hydrogen phtalate (CAP) has been investigated *in vivo*.

Indeed, only CAP shows a low enough buffer capacity to gel effectively in the cul de sac of eye. This cellulose derivative in dispersion starts to dissolve at a pH of about 5.0 as shown in Figure 7. The CAP latex containing the active compound (pilocarpine) adsorbed partially onto the surface of the polymer particles is shown in Figure 8.

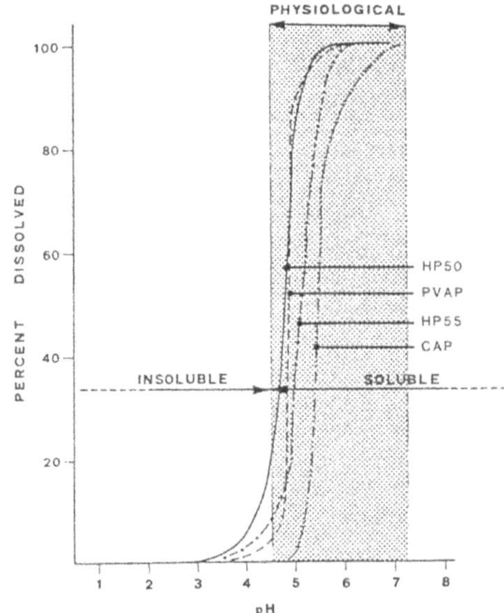

Figure 7
Solubility Profiles
of some Polymers

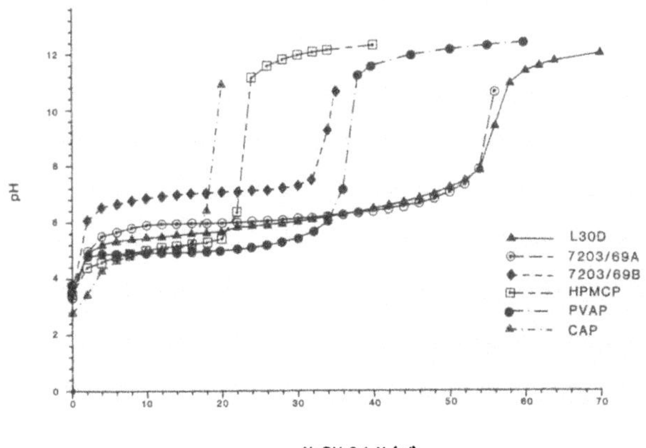

Figure 8
Neutralization Profiles for some Polymers

The latex, as shown in Figure 8 (left side), coagulates within a few seconds when placed in the cul de sac since the lacrymal fluid has a pH of 7.2. The pH of the ungelled formulation is 4.4 and is therefore sufficient to keep the dispersion in a stable form. The pH change of 2.8 units after instillation due to the surrounding tear fluid leads to an almost instantaneous transformation of the highly fluid latex into a viscous gel. The partially gelified polymeric dispersion (Figure 8, right side) shows the surface of the latex particles starting to dissolve. They cannot be washed out of the cul de sac by the lacrymal fluid and they form a microreservoir in situ with a high viscosity. This viscosity change can be simulated for an experimental polymeric dispersion (5% solid content) as shown in the same figure where it is clearly shown that a jump of 2 pH units will increase viscosity dramatically (Gurny (1983)).

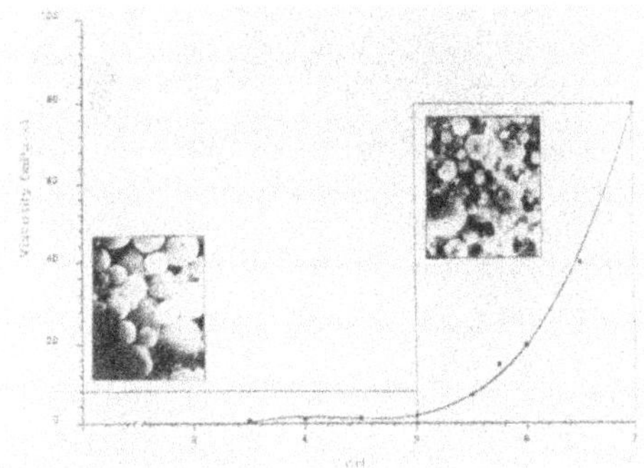

Figure 9
Viscosity Behavior of a Diluted CAP Latex
(5% Solid Content) at Various pH Values

RESULTS AND DISCUSSION

First *in vivo* results have been obtained with such *in situ* gel forming systems. The long-acting latex, once coagulated, has no impact on vision. The relative miotic response over time of such a therapeutic system with 4% pilocarpine hydrochloride in comparison to an isotonic solution is given in Figure 10.

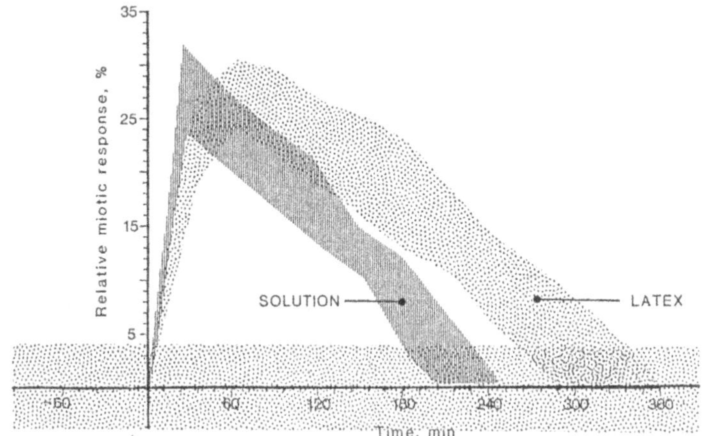

Figure 10
Comparison of the Miotic Response of Two Dosage Forms both Containing 4% Pilocarpine HCl with Indication of Noise Level and Standard Deviations

The latex formulation tested has a total content of polymer (CAP) of 30% wt/wt, an average viscosity of 50 mPa·s and an average particle size of 250 nm with a polydispersity index of 2.

Several pharmacokinetic parameters have been proposed to characterize long-acting formulations, such as the width of the miotic response peak at half the height ($\Delta_{1/2}$) (Meier (1978)), the time between the increase in activity of more than 10% ($t_{>10\%}$) and the mean residence time of activity (MRT) (Yoshida et al. (1975)). A complete analysis comprising the values for the area under curve (AUC), the maximum response intensities (RI_{max}) and the time to peak values (t_{max}) for a number of ophthalmic formulations is given in Table 3.

Preparation No		AUC	RI_{MAX}	t_{MAX}	$\Delta_{1/2}$	$t_{\Delta 10\%}$	MRT
1	Isotonic solution (4%)	3396	27	28	132	155	130
2	Poloxamer gel 25% polymer	4493	28	48	164	199	156
3	Latex system (4%)	5214	27	49	198	229	189
4	Adsorbocarpine (4%)	3534	27	32	133	159	125
5	Ophthalmic rod (950 mg (Hässle))	3199	28	58	112	141	97

Table 3
Bioavailability for Several Long Acting Formulation

The polymeric dispersion containing 4% pilocarpine (preparation No. 3) shows a substantial increase in bioavailability (AUC) as compared to the solution (increase in bioavailability by a factor of 1.5). Only the system with a sol-gel transition temperature in the range of 30°C (preparation No. 2) shows a similar result. Most commercially available formulations show no marked difference from our reference preparation No.1. By analyzing the MRT values, similar conclusions can be drawn. The response intensity is similar in all cases, whereas the appearance of the peak is delayed with formulation No. 3.

CONCLUSION

For ophthalmic use, polymeric dispersions based on the mechanism of drug adsorption onto the surface of the polymeric particles (0.3 µm average particle size) which show good biocompatibility and form a gel *in situ* after application have shown the best bioavailability increase as compared to a solution. These formulations have low viscosity and can accommodate a solid content up to 30% wt/wt. The unique feature is that they can be applied as easily as eye drops, which will result in good patient compliance. In the case of pilocarpine-containing systems, two daily instillations should be sufficient, compared to 4 to 6 applications with ordinary eye drops.

The thermosetting systems based on poloxamer 407 also show an increase in bioavailability. They present some problems with blurring of the vision and should therefore be used only during the night.

REFERENCES

BASF Wyandotte Corp., Technical Data 0S796.

Eldridge JE, Ferry JD (1954) Studies of the cross-linking process in gelation gels. J Phys Chem 58: 975-992.

Gurny R, Taylor D (1980) Development and evaluation of a prolonged acting drug delivery system for the treatment of glaucoma. In: Rubinstein MH (ed.): Proceedings of the International Symposium of the British Pharmaceutical Technology Conference, London, Solid Dosage Research Unit, Liverpool.

Gurny R (1981) Preliminary study of prolonged acting drug delivery system for the treatment of glaucoma. Pharm Acta Helv 56: 130-132.

Gurny R (1983) Latex systems. In: Breimer DD, Speiser P (eds): Topics in pharmaceutical sciences. Elsevier Science Publishers, Amsterdam; pp. 130-132.

Heilman K (1978) Therapeutische Systeme. Georg Thieme Verlag, Stuttgart.

Miller SC, Donovan MD (1982) Effect of poloxamer 407 gels on the miotic activity of pilocarpine nitrate in rabbits. Int J Pharm 12: 147-152.

Vadnere M, Amidon G, Lindenbaum S, Haslam JL (1984) Thermodynamic studies on the gel-sol transition of some pluronic polyols. Int J Pharm 22: 207-218.

Vanderhoff JW, El-Aasser MS, Ugelstad J (1979) Polymer emulsification process. U.S. Patent 4,177,177, December 4.

SEMIOLOGY OF THE TEAR FILM

M. Rolando

Department of Ophthalmology, University of Genova, Italy

Tear film changes are one of the most common problem in general Ophthalmic practice as they can be primary, but more often are the consequence of almost any affection of the ocular surface.

Their detection and understanding will indicate the correct therapeutic approach and lead to a quick benefit to the patient.

The recognition of Tear film pathology apart from cases of apparent dryness can be quite difficult. Sijögren (1933) stated that clinically many subjects with the Sicca Sindrome showed a wet eye surface. Scherz and Coll. (1974) have demonstrated that the tear volume of eyes with Keratoconjunctivitis sicca (KCS) is only 25% less than those of normal eyes.

Although it is tradition to consider each of the three layers of the tear film separately, any change in one of the tear film constituents will affect the film as a whole.

The first step for recognizing that a tear film change is present is to realize that many times when we see a red eye a tear film pathology IS present (THINK DRY EYE !).

ANAMNESIS

The anamnestic investigation can give useful hints.
The following conditions can be related to a diminished or altered tear production:

- systemic hormonal changes;
- collagen and autoimmune diseases (rheumatism, systemic Lupus Eritematosus, etc);
- dermatologic diseases (Rosacea, hyperseborrea);
- continuative use of antihistamine, beta-bloking or atropine like drugs;
- hyponutrition or surgically induced Hypovitaminosis A;
- trauma or recurrent bacterial or viral infections of the ocular surface;
- prolonged use and abuse of ophthalmic preparations containing preservatives;
- a non specified contact lens intolerance.

SUBJECTIVE SYMPTOMS

In the early phases of the disease the subjective symptoms can be

Ophthalmic Drug Delivery. Biopharmaceutical, Technological and Clinical Aspects.
M.S. Saettone, G. Bucci, P. Speiser (eds.) Fidia Research Series, vol. 11, Liviana Press, Padova

sometimes misleading; the most frequent are:
- burning, caused by the hypertonic shift of the tear film; tearing(!!) Tear film break-up due to atmospheric and environmental agents like wind, low relative humidity, smog, air conditioning can induce reflex tearing as defense.
- difficulty in opening the eyes at the wake-up, because of the poor lubrification at night.
- mucus secretion and discharge, which indicate the instability of mucus layer.

In advanced conditions more typical signs are added, which can lead to the diagnosis more easily, they are:
- foreign body sensation, which is the result of the lack of lubrification;
- dryness;
- photophobia, because of light scattering induced by cornea surface irregolarities;
- pain, because of epithelial break-down;
- vision disturbances, caused by irregular astigmatism.

OBSERVATION

Skin.
In a suspect patient the skin of the chin and of the forehead should be inspected to find signs of rosacea or sebaceous gland malfunctions which will affect the lipid layer.

Blinking dynamics.
A low "rithm" of blinking is present in Basedow patients, subjects with corneal hypoesthesia, contact lens wearers and in chronic inflammatory and neoplastic pathologies of the lid. An increased "rithm" of blinking apart from neurologic blefarospasmus is sometimes present as a defence mechanism in eyes with tear hyposecretion. Normal binking rithm is 16.8 $\pm$ 2.7 blink/min. (Abelson, 1977). In normal subjects only 80% of the blinks are complete, while 20% are incomplete or just a twich.
The frequency of incomplete blinks increases during reading or watching T.V. and whenever attention is increased.
In some individuals blinking is always incomplete, except for forced blinking, leaving an area of the eye surface uncovered by the lids (lid lag).
Bad blinking habits prevent a good spreading of the different part of the tear film and will induce tear film instability.

Hyperemia distribution.
A localized hyperemia involving the lower 2/3 of the ocular surface, while leaving the unexposed (under the lid) area normal, is probably linked to the evaporation rate and osmolarity which are increased in tear film diseases and is a sign of paramount importance for a early diagnosis (Gilbard & Coll., 1978; Rolando & Coll., 1983).

SLIT-LAMP EXAMINATION

The LID MARGIN has to be carefylly observed to look for the presence of lipid changes and Meibomianitis. A mild compression on the

Meibomian glands (applyng a Q-tip from the skin side) will give informations about trasparence, viscosity and other qualities of the Meibomian secretions.

An increased REFLECTIVITY of the conjunctival surface is associated to a globet cell loss and to the presence of epithelium squamous metaplasia characteristic of the eye surface in dry eyes.

The presence of PARTICULATE MATTER and debris on corneal surface indicate a reduction of the washing capability of the tears and are often associated to an unstable mucus.

TEAR MENISCUS hight and regularity can provide interesting informations. Normal tear meniscus is usually 0.2- 0.5 mm.. In tear film pathology tear meniscus is often scanty and shows mucus precipitates floating on its surface.
An immoble tear meniscus has to be ruled out in cases of normal thickness. The absence of movement is a sign of poor tear escretion from the puncta and the abundance of fluid is not the consequence of a normal tear production.

FLUORESCEIN can be used to stain and evidentiate the tear fluid. Fluorescein stains the fluid of intercellular spaces and the staining of the cornea or of the conjuctiva indicates an advanced damage to the ocular surface epithelium. A punctate epithelium keratopathy of the conjunctiva and of the cornea in the interpalpebral fessure, suggests either a lack of tear secretion or an increased tear evaporation.

Fluorescein staining can also be used to evidentiate the BLACK LINE. When fluorescein is applied to the tear film, using a blue cobalt light, a regular thinning of the film can be observed near the tear meniscus, in normal eyes (back line). The width of the black line is correlated to tear volume: a large and irregular black line is a sign of reduced tear volume on the eye surface.

ROSE BENGALA stains mucus, degenerated and dead cells, its use is of outmost importance to quantify the eye surface involvment and to evidentiate mucus conditions in course of tear film diseases. It is noteworth that in normal eyes a constant turnover of epithelial cells is always present and a mild Rose Bengala positivity has therefore to be considered normal.

BREAK-UP TIME (BUT) measurement can be very useful in clinical practice to demonstrate an unstable tear film.
When 1% fluorescein is applied to the temporal conjunctiva it will stain the tear film in green. The interval between the last blink and the development of the first randomly distributed dry spot (which will appear black) is defined as the BUT. In normal eyes it ranges between 15" and 45". A BUT shorter than 10" has to be considered abnormal. A BUT consistently localized in the same corneal area indicates a significant surface abnormality.
As the BUT in normals varies following the different testing settings, its reproducibility has been put into discussion. The use of fluorescein with preservatives, the size of the interpalpebral fissure, the relative humidity and the temperature of the envi-

ronment, the air movement around the eye and the characteristics of the last blink, are parameters which, if changed, will induce different results (Vanley & Coll., 1977).
To limit the influence of some of these parameters a simple instrument has recently been developed , which allows BUT measurements in more standardized conditions. This instrument consists of a dome with Placido rings that are mirrored on the tear film. The regularity of the mirrored rings can be observed through a biomicroscope. A break of the shape and of the regularity of the rings indicates the break up of the tear film.
No fluorescein is needed, the air movement is reduced by the protection provided by the dome and the size of the interpalpebral fissure can be monitored during the observation (Fig. 1).

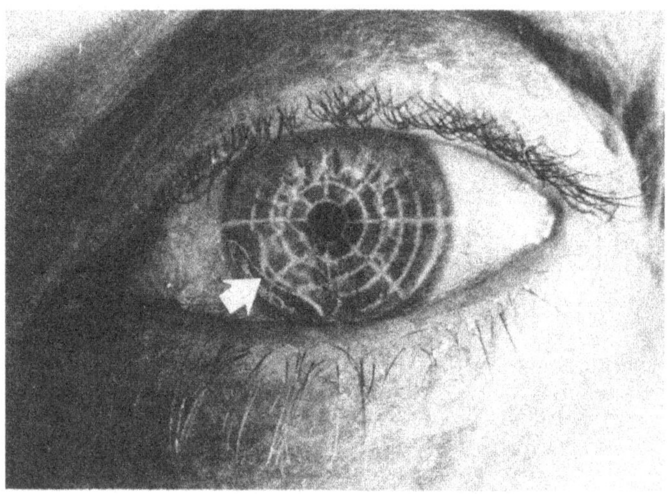

Fig. 1 - The arrow indicates a mayor break-up area of tear film as it can be seen through the instrument.

QUANTITATIVE TESTS

Shirmer I test.
This test as often been questioned because of its poor reproducibility, however it remains the only low cost system to evaluate tear production in the clinic.
The test consists in introducing a filter paper strip (35 mm. long and 5 mm. wide with 5 mm. head folded) into the outer third of the inferior fornix. The eye has to be kept open for 5', at the end of this period the lenghth of the paper wet will give the rate of tear secretion (basal + reflex).
A tentative of standardization of the Schirmer test by Von Bijsterveld showed that a value lower than 5.5 mm. in 5' has the best chance of detecting a dry eye.
The variability of the test seems to be due to different characteristics of the paper (pores size, superficial tension), to different

tear viscosities and to environmental conditions of testing (Holly & Coll., 1982-83).
Testing with eyes closed will reduce inter and intra individual variability (probably reducing the reflex tears quote).

Basal Secretion Test.
This test uses the same paper strip and procedures as for the Schirmer I, except for the fact that a drop of topical anaesthetic is instilled some minutes before testing. Normal values range over 15 mm. in 5', values under 3 - 5 mm. can be considered pathological. The concept that conjunctival and corneal anaesthesia should prevent reflex tearing is only theoretical. It has been demonstrated that the stimulation of the lid lashes, as it happens by using the Schirmer paper strip, can stimulate a reflex tearing, is able to increase the tear turnover (Jordan & Baum, 1980).

Cotton Thread Method.
More recently a new system of tear production measurement, which uses a thin cotton thread in place of the paper strip, has been introduced (Kurihashi, 1978). The head of the thread is stained with fluorescein for 5 mm.. The stained end of the thread is inserted under the outer third of the superior lid and the measurement of the wet portion is recorded after 30". The wet part of the thread appears coloured in yellow and is usually longer than 25 mm. in normals.
What this test really measures is questionable, since it seems that in such a short time the thread wetting could be just the result of the tear fluid contained in the superior fornix and meniscus.
The test however is rapid and quite reproduceable, qualities that make it interesting for clinical use.

Tear Film Turn-over.
Tear film turnover can be studied at the slit lamp using a Wood light. The time necessary to demonstrate the disappearance of a 2% fluorescein eye drop from the upper meniscus can indicate the tear turn-over time. In normal secreting eyes this is about 15' - 18'. Fluorophotometry allows a more accurate testing of tear turn-over (normal values are about 16% / min.) (Jordan & Baum, 1980).

Dilution Test.
This is a useful variation of tear turn-over test and consists in the instillation of a solution containing equal parts of 1% Fluorescein and 1% Rose Bengal. This solution will color in red the tear film. Newly secreted tears dilute the solution that will change color toward orange and yellow. In normal eyes the tear film is yellow within 5'. A much longer time is needed in cases of tear hyposecretion (Norn, 1965).

Tear Evaporation Test.
Water evaporation from the tear film is regulated by the lipid layer. Any quantitative or qualitative change of the tear film able to affect the formation, the thickness and the spreading of a normal oily layer will increase the tear water evaporation rate.
An instrument able to measure the tear evaporation rate in physiolo-

gical, non invasive and reproduceable setting has been developed in 1983 (Rolando & Refojo, 1983). This instrument indirectly gives informations about the stability of the whole tear film (BUT is related just to the precorneal film).

Normal tear films shows a water evaporation rate of 4.07 $\pm$ 0.4 .10-7 g. cm.^{2} sec-1 at the environmental conditions provided by the instrument (t=23°C; RH=30%).

Values higher than 6 $\pm$ 1.02 are constantly present in eyes with tear film instability (Rolando & Coll., 1983).

Such in higher tear evaporation rate, if not balanced by an adequate tear fluid production will result in the characteristic increase in tear osmolarity of the eyes with KCS (Gilbard & Coll., 1978).

Lysozime Concentration Test.

Lysozime is a proteine provided of bacteriolitic action produced by the main and accessory lacrimal glands. Lysozime tear fluid concentration can be used as an indicator of tear production. It has been suggested that the measurement of its concentration is more accurate than the Schirmer Test in detecting early and questionable dry eyes (Mackie & Seal, 1981). The E.L.I.S.A. technique seems to be the most reliable , in the past immuno assay or lysoplate technique have been used (Bonavida & Sapse, 1968).

Lysozime concentration in tears decreases with age at the rate of 0.01 g/1 /year after the age of 40 (Mc Gill, 1985).

The complexity of the technique makes this test rather unpractical in the clinic.

Lactoferrin Concentration Test.

Like lysozime, Lactoferrin is a protein secreted by the acinar components of the lacrimal glands with bactericide action. Lactoferrine concentration varies with age in a fashion correlable to lysozime and it is reduced in case of tear flow reduction.

Radial immuno diffusion technique is a simple, reliable and quite inexpensive system for measuring its concentration in the clinic (Janssen, 1983).

QUALITATIVE TESTS

Tear Osmolarity Measurement.

The knowledge of tear film osmolarity is particularly important in Keratoconjunctivitis sicca (KCS) because it has been hypotized that epithelial damage is a consequence of its increase (Gilbard & Coll., 1978). Tear film osmolarity is the result of the equilibrium between tear secretion and tear evaporation rates. In KCS where tear evaporation rate is increased its value is superior to 312 mOsm/1 (normal values 304 $\pm$ 10.4 mOsm/1).

The tear Osmolarity measurement unfortunately requires a specialized and costly equipment.

Tear pH Meaurement.

An increased tear pH has been found in the tear film of patients with Rosacea. Direct measurement using a mycroprobe gives pH values of 7 $\pm$ 0.2 (Abelson & Coll., 1981).

For its property of changing color at different pH, 1ul bromotimol eye drops have been used to test tear film pH. After the instillation of the drop different colours of the tear film will correspond to different pHs (Norn, 1968).

Tear Proteins Determination.
SDS polyacrilamide electrophoresis and radial immuno-diffusion techniques are the most ferquently used. As we have already seen, the knowledge of the concentration of the different proteins of the tear film can provide useful hints for assessing the cause of tear film instability (Gachon & Coll., 1982; Liotet, 1984).

Mucus Content.
A semi-quantitative test for assessment of mucus content of the tear film is the so called Dohlman test, which consists in PAS staining of the paper strip of the Schirmer test after its execution. The colour intensity of the sample indicate the mucus content of the adsorbed tear fluid and can be compared to normal or other comparison samples.

Mucus Morphology.
Mucus morphology on the eye surface can be studied in vivo by means of the Adams test (1979). The test implies the compression of the glossy part of a millipore filter on the anaesthetized surface of bulbar or tarsal conjunctiva. After PAS and Mayer ematossiline staining, mucus distribution can be observed by light mycroscopy. In normal eyes the mucus is evenly spread in form of a regular net; when tear mucus pathology is present the net is collapsed and big mucus threads appear.

Tear Mucus Ferning Test.
This test is based on the peculiar characteristics of cristallization of glycoprotein solution when they dry at room temperature. Tear samples are collected from the tears pooled in the lower fornix of the eye. Care should be taken not to grasp on the conjunctival surface. The manouvre is painless for the patient and no anaesthesia is necessary. Moreover any topical anaesthetic should be avoided because it will alterate the glicoprotein status.
The samples are allowed to dry and observed at phase-contrast light mycroscopy (60-100 X). Four types of mucus crystallization patterns can be observed (Fig. 2)
Types I and II are characteristic of normal eyes while type III and IV are present in 91.7% of eyes with KCS.
Ferning results from the interaction of the electrolytes with the high molecolar weight proteins of the tear film. Types I and II seem to express the ideal equilibrium between glycoproteins and electrolytes characteristic of the normal tear film.
The increased evaporation rate of water from the tear film present in KCS leads to an increase in electrolytes concentration in the film and to an alteration of such an equilibrium which is responsable of the bad ferning patterns of these eyes.
The test is inexpensive, simple and does not require any laboratory equipment (Rolando, 1984; Rolando & Coll., 1986).

Lipid Layer Evaluation.

The direct evaluation of the lipid layer is difficult because of the optic properties of this layer. Indirect methods however can give informations on its conditions.
Sudan red power has been used to study the limits of the lipid layer and the location of the excretory ducts of the active meibomian glands (Norn, 1980).
Color interference bands can be used to study the oily layer thickness; a red band indicate a 200 nm thick layer, the correlation between the area of the film necessary to obtain a red interference band (by reducing the lid aperture) and the area of the film at the original lid aperture can give the thickness of the lipid layer (Norn, 1979).
A very interesting Interferential Biomycroscope has been developed recently by dr. Hamano, which can evidentiate the different patterns of the lipid layer in teh different tear film conditions (Hamano & Coll., 1980).
Basing on the fact that the lipid layer regulates tear water evaporation, the overall stability an function of the whole lipid layer can be indirectly studied by means of the Tear Evaporimeter (Rolandc & Refojo, 1983).

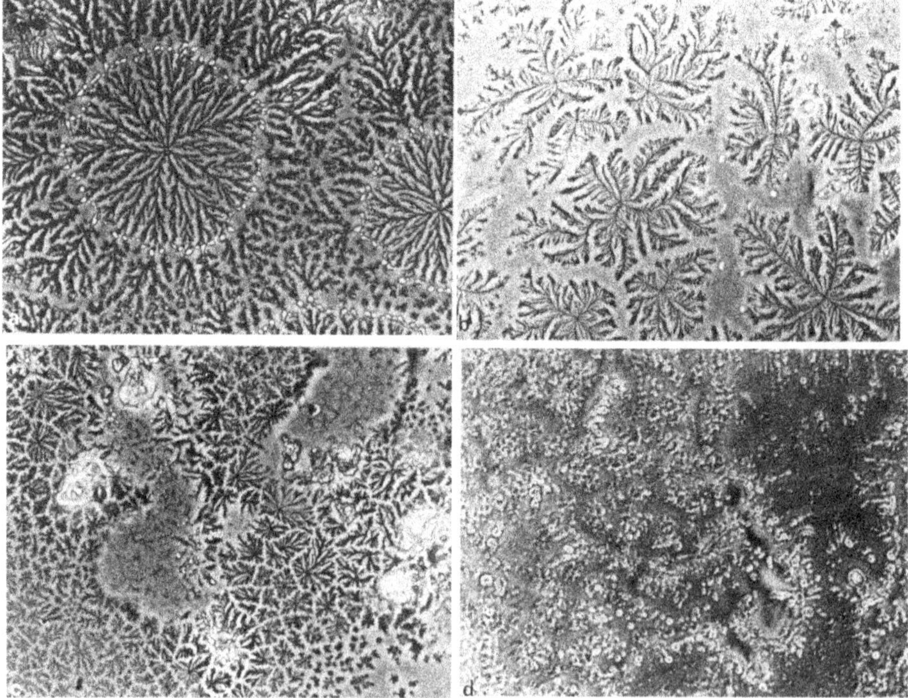

Fig. 2 - Classification of Fern Types:
a Type 1: uniform and closely branching arborization.
b Type 2: Single ferns are smaller and less branching is present. Empty spaces begin to appear.
c Type 3: Little ferns with almost no branches; many empty spaces.

d Type 4: Ferning is absent and clusters of mucus can be present.

Impression Cytology.

The importance of impression cytology for the evaluation of eye surface involvment in course of tear film pathologies has recently gained a widespread recognition.

The technique is very simple and consists in pressing on different locations of the eye surface a standardized millipore filter after topical anaesthesia. As a consequence a number of conjunctival epithelial cells becames adherent to the paper and can be removed from te eye surface. The sample is stained by a modified Papanicolau staining and then observed at light mycroscopy (Tsen, 1985; Royer & Coll., 1985; Rolando & Coll., 1986).

Goblet cells density, epithelial cells morphology and cytoplasm-nucleous ratio as well as the methacromic changes can be evaluated. A decreased goblet cell density and an increased cytoplasm-nucleous ratio together or not with signs of keratinization are caracteristic of KCS.

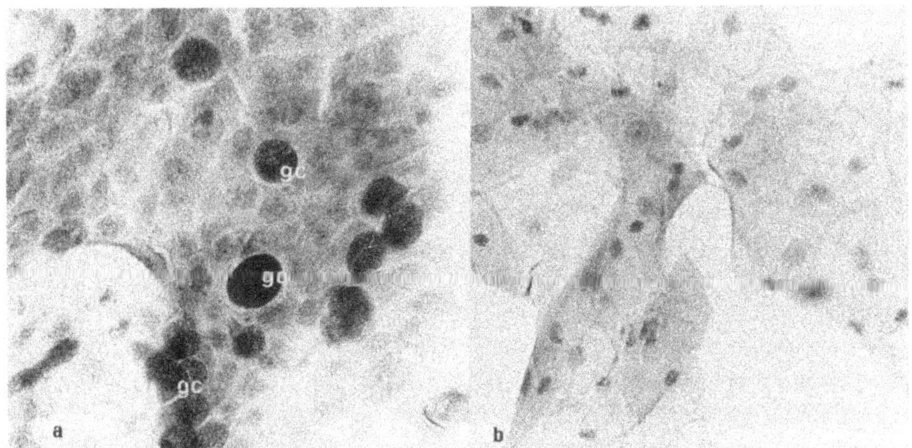

Fig. 3 - Impression Cytology:
a) Normal conjunctiva.
b) An eye with KCS shows loss of goblet cells (g.c.) and increased cytoplasm-nucleous ratio.

It is increasingly apparent that even subclinical lesions of the epithelial cell surface (e.g.loss of glycocalix) can induce or mantain tear film instability which in a vicious circle will cause epithelial cell damage and so on.

Impression cytology is furthermore the best objective system to evaluate and quantify the real efficacy of tear substitutes or other therapies in the improvement of the disease.

KEY WORDS: Tear film; Keratoconjunctivitis sicca; Eye surface.

REFERENCES

Abelson MB, Holly FJ (1977) A tentative mechanism for inferior punctate keratopathy. Am.J.Ophthalmol. 83: 866-869

Abelson MB, Udell IJ, Weston JH (1981) Normal human tear pH by direct measurement. Arch.Ophthalmol. 99: 301

Adams AD (1979) The morphology of human conjunctival mucus. Arch.Ophthalmol. 97: 730-734

Bijsterveld OP(van) (1969) Diagnostic tests in the sicca syndrome. Arch.Ophthalmol. 82: 10-14

Bonavida B, Sapse AT (1968) Human tear lysozyme.II- Quantitative determination with standard Schirmer strips. Am.J.Ophthalmol. 66: 70-76

Gachon AM, Richard J, Dastugue B (1982/83) Human tears: normal protein pattern and individual determinations in adults. Curr.Eye Res. 2: 301-308

Gilbard JP, Farris RL, Santamaria J (1978) Osmolarity of tear microvolumes in keratoconjunctivitis sicca. Arch.Ophthalmol. 96: 677-681

Gilbard JP, Carter JB, Sang DN, Refojo MF, Hanninen LA, Kenyon KR (1984) Morphologic effect of hyperosmolarity on rabbit corneal epithelium. Ophthalmology 91: 1205-1212

Hamano H, Hori M, Kawabe H et al. (1980) Clinical applications of bio differential interference microscope. Contact Intraocular Lens Med.J. 6: 229-235

Holly FJ, Lamberts DW, Esquivel ED (1982/83) Kinetics of capillary tear flow in the Schirmer strip. Curr.Eye Res. 2: 57-70

Janssen PT, Bijsterveld OP (van) (1983) A simple test for lacrimal gland functions a tear lactoferrin assay by radial immunodiffusion. Graefes Arch.Clin.Exp.Ophthalmol. 220: 171-174

Jordan A, Baum J (1980) Basic tear flow: does it exist? Ophthalmology 87:920-930

Kurihashi K (1978) Tränensekretionsmessung mit der Baumwollfadenmethode. Klin. Mbl.Augenheilk. 172: 876-879

Liotet S, Shawki D (1984) Intérêt diagnostic de l'électrophorèse des proteines lacrymales. Bull.Soc.Ophtalmol.France 84: 545-549

Mackie JA, Seal DV (1981) The questionable dry eye. Br.J.Ophthalmol. 65: 2-9

McGill J (1985) The tear film in health and disease. In: Easty DL, Smolin G(eds): External eye disease. Butterworths, London; 106-132

Mengher LS, Bron AJ, Tonge SR, Gilbert DJ (1985) A non-invasive instrument for clinical assessment of the pre-corneal tear film stability. Curr.Eye Res.4:1-7

Norn MS (1965) Tear secretion in normal eyes. Estimated by a new method: the lacrimal streak dilution test. Acta Ophthalmol. 43: 567-578

(1968) Bromothymol blue. Vital staining of conjunctiva and cornea. Acta Ophthalmol. 46: 231-242

(1979) Semiquantitative interference study of fatty layer of precorneal film. Acta Ophthalmol. 57: 766-774

(1980) Natural fat in external eye. Acta Ophthalmol. 58: 331-336

Rolando M (1984) Tear mucus ferning test in normal and keratoconjunctivitis sicca eyes. Chibret Int.J.Ophthalmol. 2(4): 32-41

Rolando M, Refojo MF (1983) Tear evaporimeter for measuring water evaporation rate from the tear film under controlled conditions in human. Exp.Eye Res. 36: 25-33

Rolando M, Refojo MF, Kenyon KR (1983) Increased tear evaporation in eyes with keratoconjunctivitis sicca. Arch.Ophthalmol. 101: 557-558

Rolando M, Baldi F, Zingirian M (1986) The effect of hyperosmolarity on tear mucus ferning. Fortschr.Ophthalmol. 83: 644-646

Rolando M, Terragna FM, Burlando S, Zingirian M (1986) La citologia ad impressione della superficie oculare in soggetti con acne rosacea. Atti 65° Congr. Soc. Oftalmol. Italiana, Siena, 1985. L.Cappelli, Bologna; pp.161-165

Royer J, Tabatabay C, Deschamps F (1985) Empreinte conjonctivale dans le syndrome de kératoconjonctivite sèche. Klin.Mbl.Augenheilk. 186: 513-514

Scherz W, Doane MG, Dohlman CH (1974) Tear volume in normal eyes and keratoconjunctivitis sicca. Graefes Arch.Clin.Exp.Ophthalmol. 192: 141-150

Sjögren H (1933) Zur Kenntnis des Keratoconjunctivitis sicca. (Keratitis filiformis bei Hypofunktion der Tränendrüsen). Acta Ophthalmol.11: suppl.2

Tseng SCG (1985) Staging of conjunctival squamous metaplasia by impression cytology. Ophthalmology 92: 728-733

Vanley GT, Leopold IH, Gregg TH (1977) Interpretation of tear film breakup. Arch. Ophthalmol. 95: 445-448

IMPRESSION CYTOLOGY OF THE BULBAR CONJUNCTIVA: POSSIBLE OBJECTIVE METHOD TO EVALUATE THE TREATMENT OF SICCA SYNDROME WITH HYALURONIC ACID

J.G. Orsoni

Institute of Ophthalmology, University of Parma, Italy

Impression cytology of the conjunctiva is a simple, repeatable, non invasive method which permits the study of conjunctival cells and offers therefore an objective way to study the functional state of the conjunctiva.

The interest of ophthalmologist to ophthalmic cytology is increasing and it is documented by the articles appearing in the American, French and German literature (1, 2, 3). Historically the interest in conjunctival cells started with Thygeson in 1946 (4) who adopted the Scraping method, after him Duszynski (5) used a cotton swab, and Norn (6) a pipette. Thatcher (7) in 1977 used an impression plastic disc and in the same year Egbert, Lauber and Maurice (8) employed first a cellulose acetate filter (Millipore) which was pressed on the conjunctiva and after pressed on a glass slide and coloured. Tseng (1) in 1984 classified the squamous metaplasia of the dry eye by the impression cytology. In Italy this method was first introduced by Rolando in 1985 (9).

Techniques used before 77' have some disadvantages; in fact scraping is uncomfortable even with local anesthesia and cannot be quickly repeated; with the cotton swab many cells are lost within the swab; the pipette method of Norn is difficult even in experienced hands; the plastic disc is uncomfortable. On the contrary impression citology with Millipore is simple, repeatable, comfortable for the patient and permits the study of a lot cells.

In dry eye syndrome the lack of tears provoques some morphological changes on the conjunctival epithelium. As previously mentioned, Tseng classified the stages of squamous metaplasia, which is the end stage of severe dry eyes, as follows:

stage 0-1: normal epithelium is present with goblet cells and small epithelial cells;

Ophthalmic Drug Delivery. Biopharmaceutical, Technological and Clinical Aspects.
M.S. Saettone, G. Bucci, P. Speiser (eds.) Fidia Research Series, vol. 11, Liviana Press, Padova © 1987

stage 2: goblet cells disappear, epithelial cells begin separating and enlarging;

stage 3: more than stage 2;

stage 4: epithelial cells markedly enlarged, separated, early keratinization;

stage 5: increased keratinization

As we have seen, Tseng considered

1) the number of goblet cells;

2) the nucleo-cytoplasm ratio in non-goblet cells;

3) the presence of keratinized cells.

We modified this classification as consequence of the observation that goblet cells are always present in cubic and cylindric epithelia and never are observed in a flat, keratinized epithelium. Therefore the reduction in number of goblet cells is dependent from the type of the epithelium. According to Tseng the N/C ratio is in normal situation 1/1 and in the stage 5 it is 1/8. We think that this observation is correct, but not very significant unless it is correlated with the type of the epithelium.

In fact cells elevated N/C ratio, basophilic cytoplasm and poor number of goblet cells correspondant to a cubic epithelium, on the contrary low N/C ratio and keratinized cytoplasm correspondant to squamous epithelium.

As consequence of those observations we decided to classify the conjunctival cells as follows:

- cubic
- cylindric
- non keratinized flat
- flat keratinized

because, as seen before, the type of epithelium includes in itself both the N/C ratio and the presence or absence of goblet cells.

PATIENTS AND METHOD

The aim of our study was to verify with impression cytology the efficacy of hyaluronic acid drops in patients affected by sicca syndrome. This type of study was already done in xerophthalmia due to avitaminosis A by Wittpenn (11), but no study exists in the literature with therapeutic agents for sicca syndrome. We felt this necessity after different studies about different products for dry eye. In fact we noted that such patients, who are psycologically very impressible, are terribly happy to have "new drops" (and it is even better if such drops are difficult or impossible to find on the market). Those patients refer to be much better subjectivally even if the objective situations is the same, or worse.

Therefore we felt the necessity of having a true objective test, as cytology is. In an open study we examined 11 patients, 10 women and 1 man, aged 40-60, who were submitted to a complete ophthalmological examination. Schirmer test was in all patients 5 mm. in 5 minutes or less. But lower as 5 seconds. The patients were controlled before the study (time 0), after 15 days (time 1) and after 30 days (time 2). At each control the following parameters were evaluated: (table 1).

TABLE 1

Fluorescein (+ or -)
Schirmer I (mm/5')
BUT (minutes)
Foreign body sensation (0 to 3)
Burning (0 to 3)
Photophobie (0 to 3)
Cytology
Photo and slit lamp.

Parameters examined at time O, I, II

A) subjective parameters: foreign body sensation, burning, photophobia which were scored from 0 to 3
B) objective parameters: Schirmer test I, BUT, Fluorescein. Schirmer test was evaluated in mm., BUT in minutes, Fluorescein was definded as positive or negative.
C) the cytologist, who was masked, considered the following parameters:

1. cellularity
2. cohesivity

3. goblet cells density
4. conservation of the cells.

These were scored as "high" or "low". We noted other parameters as well, which are impossible to be scored, as cytoplamic membrane morphology, nuclear abnormalities, the presence of lymphocytes, granulocytes and stroma fragments.

RESULTS.

These results of mentioned parameters are exposed in table II.

PTS.	SEX	AGE	SCHIRMER		BUT		FLUO		BURN.	FB.	PHOT.	
			TO	T2	TO	T2	TO	T2	TO	T2	TO	T2
R.G.	M	61	5	5	5	5	1	0	2	0	4	2
C.P.	F	62	5	4	6	6	1	0	2	0	2	0
L.V.	F	79	4	20	3	4	1	0	2	0	2	0
E.G.	F	61	10	10	7	8	1	0	3	1	2	0
L.F.	F	54	0	0	0	1	1	1	2	0	3	2
M.M	F	51	0	0	0	0	1	1	4	1	4	2
M.G.	F	58	0	0	5	5	1	0	1	0	3	0
I.M.	F	57	5	8	4	4	0	0	2	0	3	0
A.P.	F	52	6	6	7	6	1	0	2	0	0	0
M.S	F	41	2	3	9	9	1	0	3	0	1	0
F.S.	F	74	2	1	3	3	1	0	2	0	1	0

TO = time 0
T2 = time 2
BURN = burning
FB = foreign body
PHOT = photophobia

COMMENT.

Foreign body sensation and photophobia improved with good significance ($p < 0.05$), as well as fluo test considered from time 0 to time 2.

We didn't consider time 1, because no significance was demonstrated between time 0 and time 1. Concerning cytology the cells were in a significantly better state of conservation ($p < 0.05$) at time 2 as in time 0.

The morphological changes are well observed in figure 1, figure 2 respectively before and after treatment.

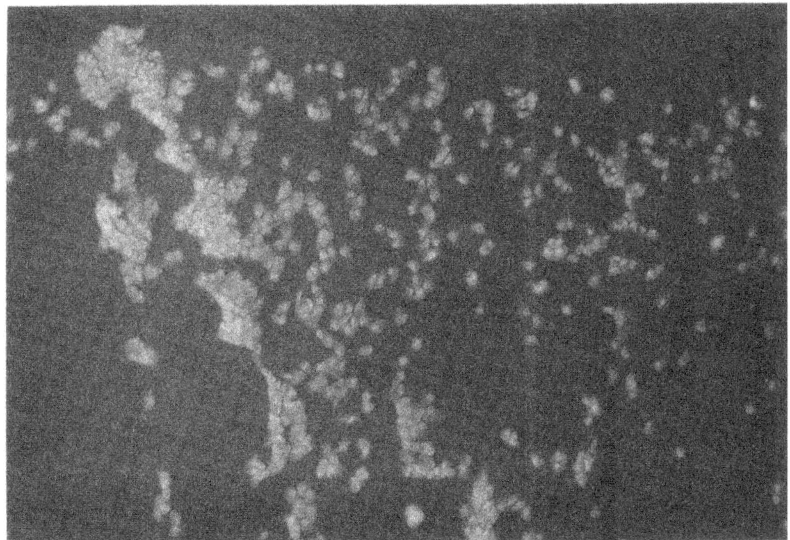

Fig. 1 Scattered cells before treatment.

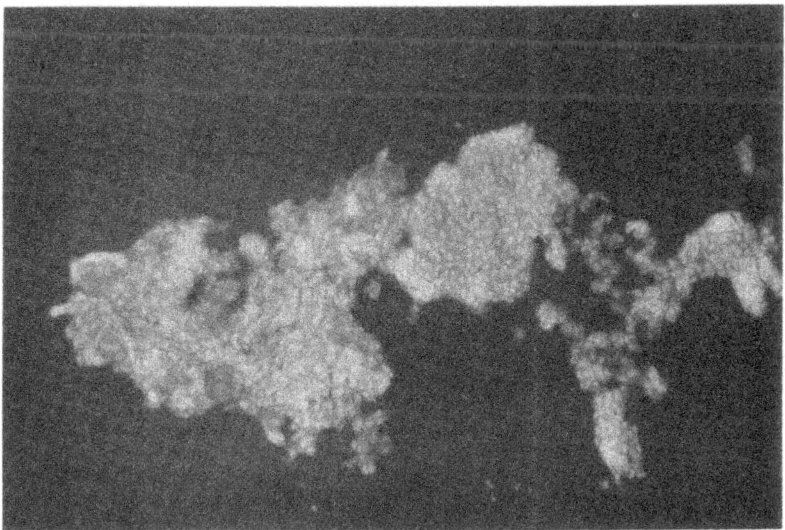

Fig. 2 Good cohesion of cells, after treatment.

This results are encouraging, but it is important to remember that it was an open study. We are studing now a group of patients a double blind trial and testing the objective of the cytological examination with a computerizde microscope.
By those two other studies we hope to confirm such promising results.

BIBLIOGRAPHY

1. Scheffer C.G. Tseng: Staging of conjunctival squamous metaplasia by impression cytology. Ophthalmology 92: 728-733, 1985
2. J. Royer, C. Tabatabay, F. Deschamps: Empreinte conjonctival dans le syndrome de kératoconjonctivite sèche. Klin. Mbl. Augneheilk., 186: 513-514, 1985
3. F.E. Kruse, J.W. Rohen, M.I. Gotz, W. Jager, W. Schimtz: Die impressioncytologie der Bindehant. Eine nichinvasive Untersuchungs methode. Ophthalmologie, 83 Tagung der dog, Springer 1986.
4. Thygeson P.: The cytology of conjunctival exsudates. Am. J. Ophthalmol. 29, 1499, 1946
5. Duszynski L.: Cytology of the conjunctival sac. Am. J. Ophthalmol. 37, 576, 1954
6. Norn MS: Cytology of the conjunctival fluid. Acta Ophthalmol. 59, suppl. 11, 1960
7. R.W. Thatcher, S. Darougar, B.R. Jones: Conjunctival impression cytology. Arch. Ophthalmol. 95, 678-681, 1977
8. Egbert P.R., Lauber S., Maurice D.M.: A simple conjunctival biopsy. Am. J. Ophthalmol. 84, 798-801, 1977
9. Rolando M.: Citologia ad impressione della congiuntiva: una biopsia incruenta - Bollettion di oculistica - Atti 1985
10. J.R. Wittpenn, Scheffer C.G. Tseng, A. Sommer: Detection of early xerophthalmia by impression cytology. Arch. Ophthalmol. 104, 237-239, 1986.

STRUCTURAL PROPERTIES OF CONTACT LENS MATERIALS

M. Casini

Gruppo di studio Carl Zeiss S.p.A.
Divisione Lenti a Contatto
Via Caldera, 21/C3, Milano, Italy

Polymer chemistry has contributed greatly to the evolution of contact lens industry. Although some contact lenses were used before the development of polymer science, the commercial availability of PMMA (polymethylmethacrylate) and p(HEMA) (2-poly-hydroxyethylmethacrylate) has facilitated the expansion of the contact lens market.
This work classifies the contact lens materials now marketed or under investigation. It also points out some important structural and physicochemical properties relevant to the use of contact lenses in the correction of ametropias, viz., the effect of the environment on dimensional stability, the absorption of solutes, oxygen permeability, and the interactions with the precorneal tear film.

INTRODUCTION

The design and development of materials for specific biomedical applications is one of the most fascinating scientific subjects now under investigation. However, it is not perhaps immediately evident that the use of polymers for contact lenses is an example of biomedical application of synthetic materials. A variety of polymeric materials widely used for hard and soft contact lenses have been discussed by Refojo (1), Tighe (2), Peppas (3), and Casini (4), among others. In most of these reviews, the properties of polymers for contact lenses are analysed and evaluated.

A chemist who has the responsibility of designing a new polymer must deal with problems concerning interactions of a synthetic macromolecular structure with biological fluids. The purpose of this work is to examine the principal structural properties of contact lens materials in connection with the above mentioned topic.

The available contact lenses have been classified by Refojo (5) as follows:

I - RIGID

1. PMMA (polymethylmethacrylate)
2. Other polymers:
   a. Cellulose Acetate Butyrate (CAB)
   b. Silicon resin
   c. Syloxane/Methacrilate
   d. Alkylstyrene

Ophthalmic Drug Delivery. Biopharmaceutical, Technological and Clinical Aspects.
M.S. Saettone, G. Bucci, P. Speiser (eds.) Fidia Research Series, vol. 11, Liviana Press, Padova © 1987

II - SEMI-RIGID

1. Fluorocarbon

III - ELASTOMERIC

1. Silicone rubber
2. Acrylic rubber

IV - SOFT HYDROPHILIC

1. Hydrogel
a. Low hydration (to 45%)
b. Medium hydration (to 55%)
c. High hydration, (to 80%)

V - BIOPOLYMERS

1. Protein
2. Collagen

The terms "hard" and "soft" contact lenses are used to classify contact lens materials according to their mechanical properties. In the above classification, however, the complex problems the chemist is faced with in designing contact lens materials are overlooked.

Recently Peppas (3), in a study of the optimization of the structure of polymers for contact lens applications, indicated that these materials, as thin films, must possess at least six basic properties: chemical, biological, optical, surface, mechanical and diffusive.

I - Rigid lenses

1. Polymethylmethacrylate (PMMA).

PMMA lenses, introduced in the late 1930's, are still widely used. The polymer is obtained with an addition polimerization of methylmethacrylate monomer (MMA) with bulk polymerization (Fig. 1): the result is a linear polymer, rigid at room temperature. The random configuration of the asymmetric carbon atoms, along with the bulky side groups, produces a highly amorphous structure endowed with a high trasparency to visible light. Various grades of "modified" PMMA are also used for contact lenses.

100% Methyl Methacrylate Monomer ---------→ Polymethyl Methacrylate (PMMA)

Fig. 1 - Polymerization process for Polymethylmethacrylate.

Most PMMA lenses consist of branched polymer, or of polymer ligthly cross-linked with dimethacrylate comonomer, or of blends of PMMA with small amounts of additives, in order to improve strength, hardness, and scratch resistance. The most frequently used crosslinking agent is ethylene glycol dimethacrylate (EGDMA): the resulting hard material has excellent machinability and durability properties, and has been used successfully for several decades as a contact lens material (Fig.2). As shown in the figure, the molecule contains mainly methyl groups and esterified carboxyl groups. The absence of suitable hydrophilic groups (such as OH, or others) in the molecule renders thi material unable to absorb water.

```
                                  CH3
                                  O
           CH3      CH3           C=O      CH3
     -CH2-C-CH2-C-CH2-C-CH2-C-CH2-
           C=O      C=O           CH3      C=O
           O        O                      O
           CH3      CH3                    CH3

                    CH3                    CH3      CH3
                    O                      O        O
           CH3      C=O           CH3      C=O      C=O
     -CH2-C-CH2-C-CH2-C-CH2-C-CH2-C-CH2-
           C=O      CH3           C=O      CH3      CH3
           O                      O
           CH3                    CH3
```

Fig. 2. Structural formula of Polymethylmethacrylate

Since the degree of hydration and the polarity of the molecule determines the oxygen permeability, a hard PMMA lens which absorbs approximatively 0.5% water has practically no oxigen permeability. Therefore, in order to maintain the corneal metabolism intact the lens must perform certain movements on the cornea, to allow an exchange of tear fluid between the lens and the cornea.

Due to the absence of polar groups on the surface (Fig.3), the material has no tendency to accumulate deposits of tear film components, protein and lipids, and to interact with preservatives. The wettability of PMMA is also poor, on account of the absence of hydrophilic groups.

```
CH3   CH3   CH3   CH3   CH3
 |     |     |     |     |
 O     O     O     O     O
 |     |     |     |     |
C=O   C=O   C=O   C=O   C=O
_|_____|_____|_____|_____|___
```

Fig. 3 - PMMA surface groups

2a. Cellulose Acetate Butyrate (CAB)

A more recent class of rigid contact lens combines some of the positive features of both PMMA and hydrogel lenses. The first study on CAB lenses was done by Stahl et al. in 1973 (6). CAB, like PMMA, is a thermoplastic resin; however, unlike PMMA it consists of naturally occurring polymeric components. The type of CAB normally used for contact lenses (7) contains about 13% acetyl groups, 37% butyryl groups, and only 2% hydroxyl groups (Fig.4).

The addition of butyrate groups tends to increase the flexibility of the polymer and its resistance to moisture. At the same time, this addition tends to decrease the hardness and resistance to greasy materials (8). Due to the presence of free hydroxyl groups, this molecule is more polar and about 30% more wettable than PMMA. Thus, it can react with other substances (9) absorb water (about 2%), and is oxygen-permeable. As CAB lenses perform relatively large movement on the cornea, it can be concluded that this type of lens produces less interference with the corneal metabolism than the PMMA lens. On the other

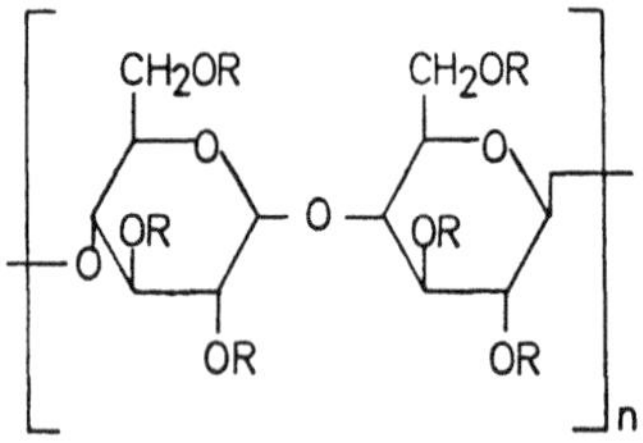

Fig. 4. Structural formula of Cellulose Acetate Butyrate.

hand, more deposits on the lens surface and a larger tendency to microbial contamination are to be expected. Due to its water content, CAB is subject to a marked hydration and dehydration cicle accompanied by changes in the lens parameters (10). This problem has been overcome by adding a copolymer, EVA (Ethylene vinyl acetate) (11) (Fig.5).

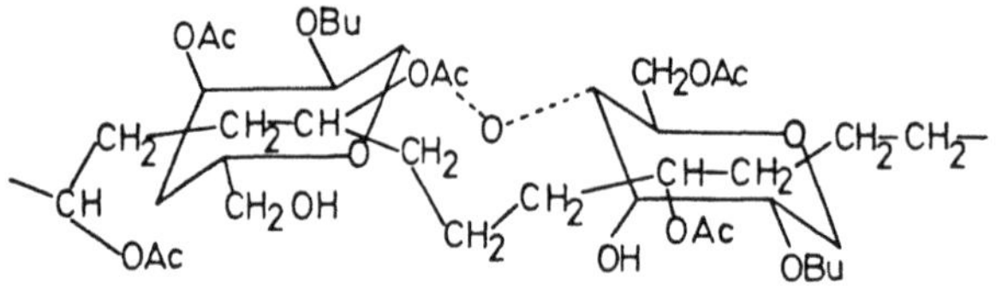

Fig.5. Structural formula of Anduran (CAB + EVA copolymer)

2b. Silicone/Acrylate copolymers

The current gas-permeable materials consist of two or more monomers that are copolymerized. The polymerization of rigid gas-permeable lenses is complex and sometimes incomplete. These lenses are made generally of copolymers of methylmethacrylate with a siloxanyl alkyl methacrylate and other monomers to enhance their oxygen permeability (Fig.6).

Siloxane monomer	+	Organic acid monomer	+	Methyl methacrylate monomer	-------→	Silicone acrylate copolymer

Fig.6. Polymerization process for silicone/acrylate lenses

The copolymer has a backbone that consist essentially of methacrylate links with side branches carrying various radicals, some with the siloxane bonds. These lenses contain silicon, not silicone. The properties of the monomer used in the polymerization process are listed in Table I.

Table I. Essential properties of the principal monomers used in silicone/acrylate copolymers

Silicone	Methacrylic acid and HEMA	Methyl methacrylate
oxygen permeability poor wettability fair mechanical & optical properties excellent oxygen permeability	poor mechanical & optical properties fair permeability excellent water affinity	mechanical and optical stability poor permeability fair wettability excellent mechanical & optical properties

The groups present in a silicone/acrylate surface are methyl ($-CH_3$), hydroxyl (-OH), carboxyl (-COOH) and siloxane segments (Fig.7):

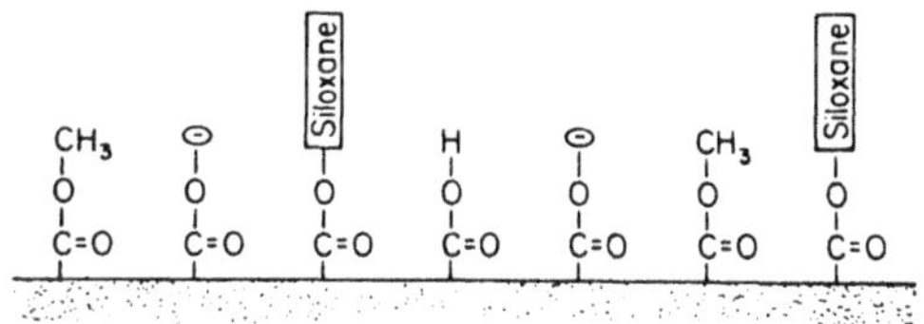

Fig.7 . Surface of a silicone/acrylate lens (12).

Each group undergoes a specific interaction with ions and preservatives in the tears and in contact lens solutions. There are three kinds of surface interactions: a) electrostatic, which create negative sites on the surface of the lens by exchanging H+ ions with ions from the surrounding solutions, thus enhancing and stabilising the wettability; b) hydrogen bonding, which enhances wettability as a result of interactions with polymers present in contact lens solutions (such as e.g.

cellulose derivatives); c) hydrophobic interactions, which produce an adverse effect by attracting hydrophobic molecules, and by binding proteins and lipids on the surface. Due to the organic acids used in the polymerization process (i.e. itaconic acid), the copolymer has a significant negative charge.

The three most important features of contact lenses made with this copolymer are: a) flexibility, b) wettability and c) oxygen permeability.

a) The flexibility depends upon the presence in the molecule chain of a flexible covalent bond such as the silicone-oxygen bond (Fig.8):

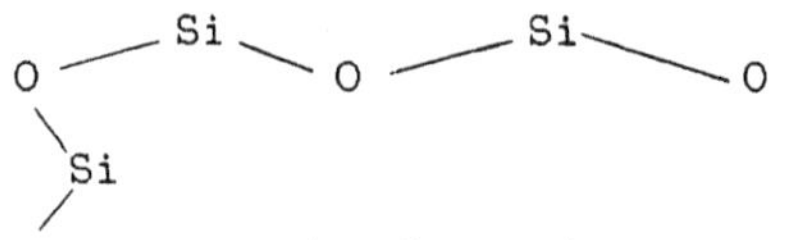

Fig.8 . Silicone-oxygen bonds produce a great flexibility.

The polymer flexibility, or mobility of the polyer chains can be reduced: 1) by increasing the crosslinking density; 2) by making the individual chains more rigid through the use of appropriate monomers; and 3) by increasing the strength of the interaction between chains, using monomers capable of strong interactions (13).

b) - Wettability. Two distinct methods can be used to increase the wettability of lens materials containing silicone, siloxanylalkyl esters or CAB: 1) surface treatment, or 2) increase of the inherent wettability of the polymer chains. In a material containing a high percentage of hydrophobic monomers, the surface treatment is accomplished by ionizing radiation, or by chemical reactions on the surface. With these processes, the hydrophobic groups on the surface are converted to hydrophilic ones. The other method, particularly used with silicon-containing contact lens materials, consists of the free radical-initiated addition of hydrophilic monomers. Thus, hydrophilic monomers are directly incorporated into the plastic material (Fig. 9):

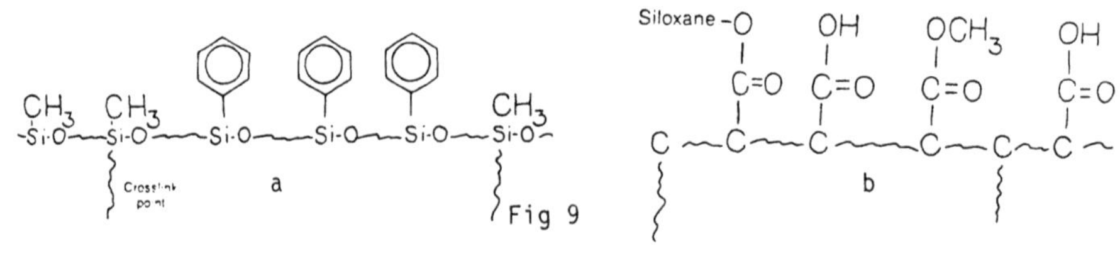

Fig. 9 - a) Silicone/acrylate material containing a high percentage of silicon-containing monomers; b) Hydrophilic monomers directly incorporated into the material (Cf. Ref. 13).

The implication of the use of one process respect to another is that in a lens treated with ionizing radiation the optical parameters cannot be modified during the fitting process.

c) - Oxygen permeability. The gas transmissibility of this class of polymers results from the special flexibility associated with the silicon-oxygen bond, and from the large spaces created between chains by bulky side groups.

2c. Styrene-based polymers

Styrene-based lenses are now manufactured by two firms (14). Pentasilcon P (15) is composed of tertiary butyl styrene copolymerized with four other monomers, one of which contains silicone to increase permeability (Fig. 10a).Since t-butyl styrene is not inherently wettable, the lenses are submitted to an appropriate surface treatment. After treatment, the silicone traces left on the lens surface are hydrolyzed off without affecting the silicone in the material itself (Fig. 10b): the end result is a hydrophilic surface.

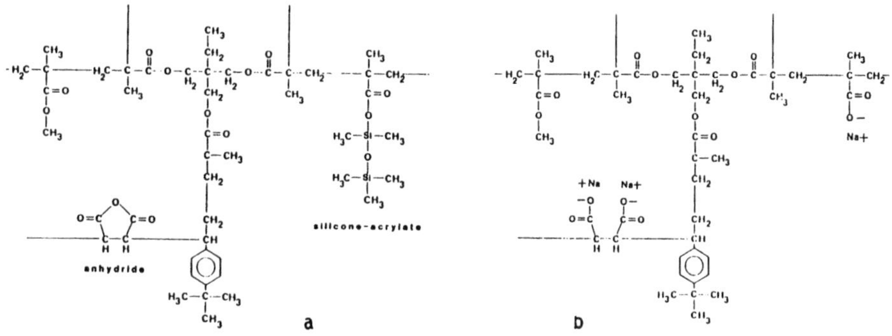

Fig. 10 - a: structural formula of Pentasilcon P. b: the material after the caustic bath: the anhydride is activated and wettability is enhanced.

Styrene is more stable than PMMA, and can be made thinner to reduce 3 and 9 o'clock striae problems. Another polymer under trial is composed of p-butyl styrene, and contains no silicone.

II - Semi-rigid lenses

Fluoropolymers

These materials were first investigated for use in contact lenses in the late sixties, with the CLP-2A Du Pont lens. All the fluoropolymer materials described in the first patents (16) consisted of acrylic polymer backbones with a fluorinated side chain (Fig. 11a). These strucures provided an improvement in oxygen permeability over PMMA, but the surfaces were non-wettable and required surface post-treatment. In the early eighties many of these problems were overcome, and today's fluoroplastics for contact lenses can be divided in two categories: a) fluoro/MMA copolymers (Fig. 11b) and b) fluoro-silicone/acrylate copolymers. The main advantage of the fluoroplastics is in their superior surface properties. The low surface tension of the fluorinated polymer unit decreases surface reactivity, thus reducing the interaction between the lens and proteins and lipids present in the tear film. This feature, combined with good oxygen transport characteristics, make these materials valid components in contact lenses for correction of ametropias.

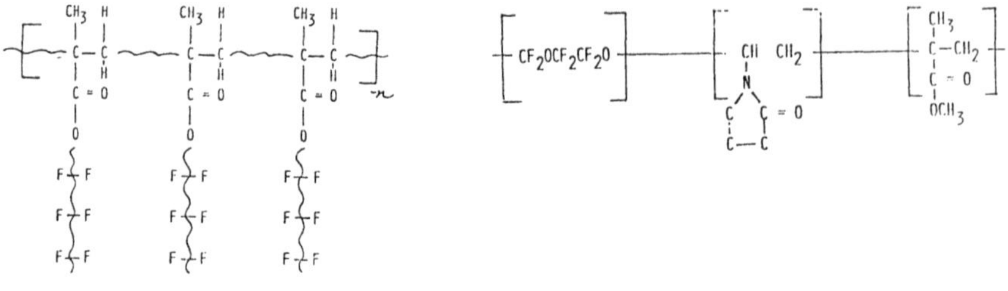

Fig. 11 - a: structure of previous fluoropolymers;
b: fluorofocon A.

The permeability of fluoroplastics is due to the solubility of gases within the material. There are fewer and/or smaller (17, 18) screen-like holes in the fluoroplastic material, thus oxygen must be absorbed from the tear film and solubilized through the lens matrix.

III Elastomeric lenses

Silicone, [poly(siloxane)].

Silicone polymers result from condensation: the final products, such as Dimefocon A (Fig.12), are used as construction materials for contact lenses.

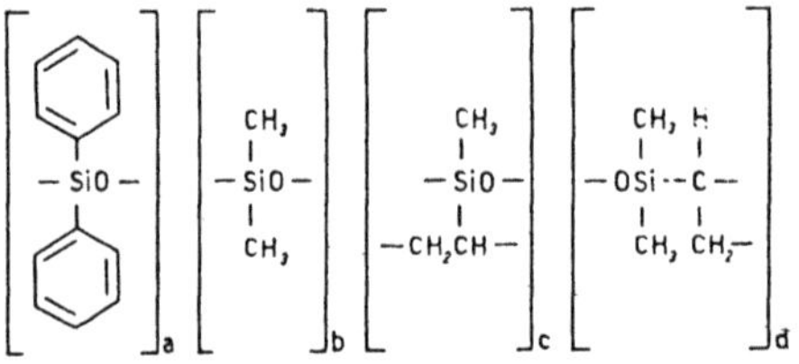

Fig.12 . Structural formula of Dimecofon A; a silicone contact lens material.

These materials are composed of silicon atoms, attached to oxygen atoms to form the siloxane bond: Si-O. This bond is part of the siloxane moiety which is repeated many times in the polymer (Fig.13):

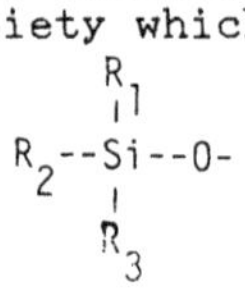

$$R_2\text{--}\underset{R_3}{\overset{R_1}{\mathrm{Si}}}\text{--}O\text{-}$$

Fig 13
The siloxane bond

Fig. 13. The siloxane bond.

Generally R is oxygen, except at the end of the molecule where it is a hydrocarbon radical; R and R are hydrocarbon radicals. The most common radicals used in contact lens silicone materials are reported in Table II:

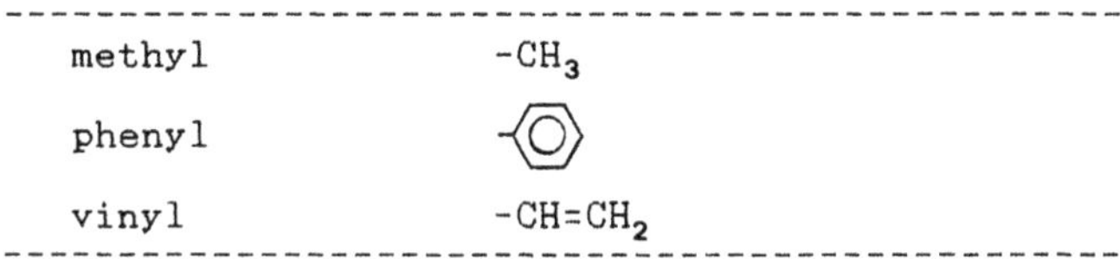

methyl	$-CH_3$
phenyl	
vinyl	$-CH{=}CH_2$

Table II. Radicals used in silicone materials

The main feature of silicones is their very high oxygen permeability, the gas being transported by diffusion through the materials (19). Another feature is their inertness. On the other hand, the surfaces are hydrophobic (contact angle between 85 to 100° C). The finished lens must therefore undergo a hydrophilization process. The inertness of silicone and the oxygen permeability are then reduced or destroyed, so the material reacts with the components of the tear film, forming very tenacious deposits.

IV Soft hydrophylic

Hydrogels.

Hydrogels are coherent, covalently crosslinked systems which form a three-dimensional network or matrix that can hold water or an aqueous solution. The polymeric network consists of repeating units of the same or of different monomers, which form long chains joined by bridges of a crosslinking compound (21). The first and most widely used soft lens consists of 2-hydroxyethylmethacrylate crosslinked with a small amount (usually less than 3%) of EGDMA (Fig.14).

The material is amorphous, and, due to crosslinking, it is a thermosetting plastic. The amount of water that a system can hold depends on the number of hydrophylic groups, and on its type; it also depends on the amount of crosslinking in the network. At a degree of about 0.1% of crosslinkage, HEMA absorbs 45% water; at 1.0, the water uptake is roughly 38%. The water uptake also depends on the presence and the amount of additional chemical compounds, like polyvinylpyrrolidone.

On the other hand polar groups that react easily are a drawback when other substances come in contact with this material. Poly(HEMA) consequently tends to accumulate deposits on the surface and favours bacterial growth. If these deposits are not removed irritation occurs.

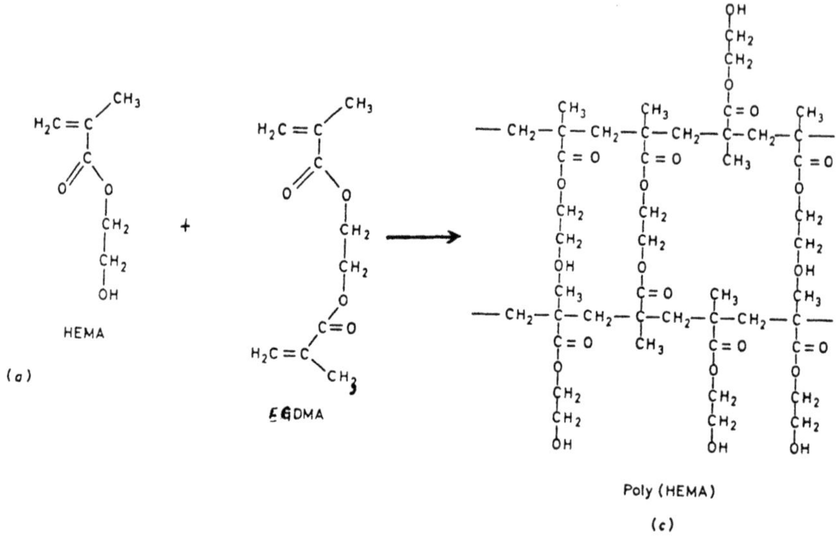

Fig.14. Hydroxyethylmethacrylate (a) and etyleneglycol dimethacrylate (EGDMA) (b); crosslinked polymer (c).

Acknowledgments

The author is grateful to Drs Tomasini and Pescosolido for thier critical review of the paper and the suggestion.

REFERENCES

1) Refojo M.F. (1984). General polymer characteristics. J. AM. Optom. Ass. 55. 184-185.

2) Tighe B.J. (1983). Contact lens materials. MOI March.

3) Peppas N.A, (1981). Properties-based optimization of the structure of polymers for contact lens applications. Contact Int. Lens Med. J. 7: 300-314.

4) Casini M.(1982). Criteri generali per lo sviluppo di nuovi materiali. AIO Atti 2, Regione Triveneto, 85-92.

5) Refojo M.F. (1985). Polymers in contact lenses: an overview. Current Eye Research 4: 719-723.

6) Stahl N.O., Ivani O. (1974). Report on laboratory studies and preliminary clinical application of a gas-permeable plastic contact lens. J. Am. Optom. Ass. 45: 302-307.

7) Kreiner C. (1980). Kontactlinsenchemie. Median-Verlag Heidelberg pp. 95-96.

8) Lowther G.E. (1983). Gas permeable rigid contact lenses. Optometry Documenta.

9) Feldman G.I. (1977). Chemical and physical properties of cellulose acetate butyrate as related to contact lenses. Contact Lens J. 11: 25-31.

10) Pearson R.M. (1975). Dimensional stability of several hard contact lens materials. Am. J. Opt. & Phy. Optics 54:826-833.

11) Germ. Offen. 2.856.891.

12) Olson A. (1986). Rigid gas permeable contact lenses, in "Polymer chemistry", Bennet E.S., Grohe R.M. (eds). Professional Press, New York; pp 77-92.

13) Olson A. (1982). Surface properties: wettability and adsorption. Contact Lens J. 10: 11-15.

14) Grieco A. (1984). Freedom choice: a gas-permeable materials overview. Int. Contact Lens Clinic. 11: 720-729.

15) U.S. Patent 4.581.184; U.S. Patent 4.243.790.

16) U.S. Patent 3.542.461; U.S. Patent 3.940. 207; U.S. Patent 3.944.347.

17) Keates R.H., Inhlenfeld J.V., Isaacson W.B. (1984). An introduction to Fluoropolymer contact lenses: a new class of materials. CLAO J. 10: 332-334.

18) Caroline P.J., Ellis E.J. (1986). Review of the mechanism of oxygen transport through rigid gas permeable lenses. Int. Eyecare 2:210-213.

19) Hwang S., Tang T.E.S., Kammermeyer K. (1971). Transport of dissolved oxygen through silicone rubber membrane. J. Macromol. Sci-Phys B5(1): 1-10.

20) Peppas N.A. (1982). Contact lenses as biomedical polymers, in: "Extended wear contact lenses for aphakia and miopia", J. Hartstein Ed, C.V. Mosby, St. Louis pp. 6-43.

CONTACT LENSES AS THERAPEUTIC SYSTEMS

G. Calabria and F. Rathschuler

Department of Ophthalmology, University of Genova, Italy

The use of contact lenses in treating conditions such as epithelial defects, corneal edema and dry eye syndromes has been extensively investigated. Contact lenses, by shielding the epithelium from the abrasive action of the lids, may avoid mechanical disruption of the ocular surface and aid its healing. Hydrophilic materials, acting as a fluid reservoir, are useful in dry eye syndromes when used in conjunction with frequent artificial tears instillation; sometimes they are also useful in mild degrees of corneal edema when applied in conjunction with hypertonic solutions.
Soft contact lenses can also be used as true ocular therapeutic systems: the ability of hydrophilic materials to imbibe and release fluids can have therapeutic implications where the use of topical ophthalmic drugs is concerned. When placed on the eye surface, lenses soaked in drug solutions have been found to produce significantly greater aqueous levels than the simple administration of the eye drops . By employing soft contact lenses as drug release system, it has sometimes been possible to reduce the drug concentration, while maintaining its effect on the eye and avoiding undesirable systemic effects.
The potential of hydrophilic lenses as vehicles for drug administration has not been well investigated. The uptake of the drug by the lens and the elution rate from the hydrogel to the target tissues may vary, depending on the lens materials and on the drug used. Drugs penetrate hydrophilic contact lenses and are eluted at a rate which depends upon the pore size between the crosslinkage of the three-dimensional structure of the hydrogel, upon concentration and molecular size of the drug and upon many other conditions.
The clinical effectiveness of contact lenses as an ocular therapeutic system is known only for some drugs used in sight-threatening ocular diseases like acute glaucoma, and in severe infections.

INTRODUCTION

Soft contact lenses contain water: the water in the hydrogel can be replaced with aqueous solutions of different ophthalmic drugs without changing the physical properties of the lens (shape, trasparency, elasticity, etc.). The therapeutic value of

Ophthalmic Drug Delivery. Biopharmaceutical, Technological and Clinical Aspects.
M.S. Saettone, G. Bucci, P. Speiser (eds.) Fidia Research Series, vol. 11, Liviana Press, Padova © 1987

soft contact lenses was first described by Sedlacek (1965): this author proved that a contact lens saturated with 1% mesocaine solution induced analgesia of the cornea more effectively and in a shorter time than the instillation of the same solution.

Waltman and Kaufman (1970) showed that hydrophilic contact lenses soaked in fluorescein produced significantly greater aqueous levels of the dye than the administration of drops. After this work, mainly in the early seventies, a great number of publications on drug release by soft contact lenses have appeared. Subsequently, with the advent of conjunctival inserts, specially designed to provide continuous ophthalmic drug delivery, studies on the use of contact lenses as therapeutic systems have decreased.

Soft contact lenses have been extensively investigated for use in ametropia and for treating epithelial defects, corneal edema and dry eye syndromes: hydrogel CL, by shielding the epithelium from the abrasive action of the lids, may avoid its mechanical disruption and facilitate its healing. In dry eye syndromes, hydrophilic contact lenses can also act as a tear substitute when soaked in artificial tears, or as a fluid depot when used in conjunction with artificial tears instillation.

Soft contact lenses can be useful in the treatment of corneal edema: the lens alone or in conjunction with a hypertonic solution instilled on the lens or preadsorbed by the lens can act by reclaiming liquids from the corneal tissue, while at the same time protecting and improving the optical quality of the ocular surface.

Soft contact lenses can also be used as true ocular therapeutic systems. However, the liberation of a drug from a contact lens depends on a great number of variables, the most important of which are the following:

1) lens characteristics: polymer properties, pore size, lens hydration, thickness and other lens dimensions;
2) drug characteristics: polymer-binding capacity, molecular weight, distribution in the lens, diffusion rate;
3) characteristics of the ocular environment: temperature, pH, tear evaporation, quality and quantity of tears, blinking frequency and lid pressure on the lens.

This list is not exaustive, but it does illustrate the difficulties involved in predicting the pharmacokinetics of drug release.

We here review the more important experimental and clinical results in the use of contact lenses as therapeutic system.

Drug diffusion across hydrogel lenses and distribution kinetics on the eye

Soft contact lenses are often used in conjunction with topical medications such antiglaucoma drugs, steroids and antibiotics. For best results, it is necessary to determine the drug permeation through the contact lens material, and the drug distribution in the eye with respect to time. It is also important to know, for every drug, the diffusion coefficient in the various hydrogel lens models.

Mc Carey et al. (1984) attemped to design a kinetic model to estimate the drug distribution on a theoretical eye covered by a hydrogel contact lens.

Mc Carey and Wilson (1982) investigated lenses with a water content ranging from 38.6% to 79.5% and a thickness ranging from

0.25 to 0.61 mm. The diffusional properties were determined for gentamicin chloride (Table I).

TABLE 1

Lens Type	Water %	Thickness				Diffusion Constants (DK) cm^2/sec
		Mean	Range	No	SD	
Sauflon	79.5*	.194	.145-.312	21	.048	$-3.2 \cdot 10^{-7}$
Permalens	68.9*	.257	.248-.270	21	.007	$-2.65 \cdot 10^{-7}$
Idrocurve II_{55}	50.5*	.112	.093-.144	21	.016	$-1.52 \cdot 10^{-8}$
CSI	40	.054	.049-.059	2	-	$-8.0 \cdot 10^{-10}$
Bauch and Lomb	38.6	.061	.060-.062	2	-	$-1.0 \cdot 10^{-10}$

* McCarey, B.E. and Wilson, L.A., 1982

The study showed that the distribution kinetics of drugs instilled as eyedrops into the conjunctival cul de sac is very complicated. There is an immediate redistribution of the drug: the action of the lids causes the drug to be diluted by newly produced tears, concentrated by tears evaporation, drained off throughout the lacrimal duct and mixed with the tears under the contact lens by a physical exchange around the edge of the lens. All the parameters were defined by a series of equations, but in practice it appeared difficult to predict the distribution kinetics of the drug (Fig. 1).

Mc Carey et al (1984) concluded that:

- the rate at which a drug can diffuse across various hydrogels is directly related to their water content;
- the flux values are affected by variables such as lens thickness and concentration gradient of solute: the main pathway for the drug distribution depends on the forced exchange of the drug and not on its molecular size or charge, or on the permeability of the hydrogel to the drug.

Therefore, the most significant parameters are tear production and contact lens fit. If these factors are altered dramatic differences are observed in the drug distribution (Figures 2 and 3).

If the normal tear production is reduced, less new tears are produced to dilute the instilled drug: the drug is thus more effective. An elevated tear production, on the other hand, results in rapid clearance of the instilled drug.

The great variability in tear production in normal and pathological conditions greatly influences the efficacy of topical therapy. The tearing eye accumulates only 4.5% of the original drug concentration when drops are given at 10 minute intervals, and only 1.6% at 30 minute intervals (Figures 4 and 5).

Altering the contact lens fit also affects the exchange of the drug under the lens; both the volume under the lens and the clearance of the lens edge are important. The smaller the posterior lens tear volume, the greater the drug accumulation under the lens.

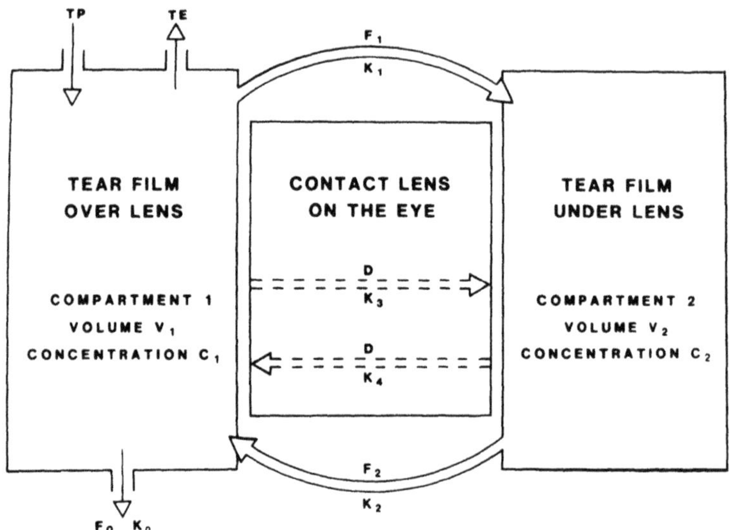

Figure 1. Kinetic model for distribution based on a two-compartment model with the contact lens as a barrier between the two compartments. (Cf. Mc Carey et al. 1984)

In conclusion, the theoretical kinetic model of Mc Carey et al. (1984) suggests that drug instillation intervals of over 30 min. are not conducive to significant drug accumulation in tears under a contact lens: a tearing eye should not have drug instillation intervals that exceed 5 minutes.

The lens is an useful tool only if it concentrates the drug from the sorrounding tear film and if it becomes a significant depot for the drug, thereby producing a different relative drug distribution. On this account, several explanations for a certain inconsistency in the efficacy of therapies based on the instillation of eyedrops on a bandage lens or on a hydrophilic contact lens are possible (Smith et al., 1982). Although recent studies have reported positive results, this method is always less reliable than the use of presoaked contact lenses.

Ellis et al. (1985) found that, following a single drop application, contact lenses did not have a significant effect on the thirty-minute concentration of the drug in the aqueous humor of the rabbit: under these conditions, contact lenses did not produce a time-release reservoir. Commercially available pilocarpine eyedrops may be used in the presence of soft contact lenses without any alteration in the observed therapeutic response.

Matoba et al. (1985) obtained data indicating that the presence of water (either 38.6% or 71%) in soft contact lenses does not hinder tobramycin delivery to the cornea and may, in fact, enhance drug availability. While the drug levels in the eyes with contact lenses were significantly different from the control eyes only at four hours, the experimental corneas had higher antibiotic levels at every time point assayed, except after one hour, in the high water content lens group (Figure 6).

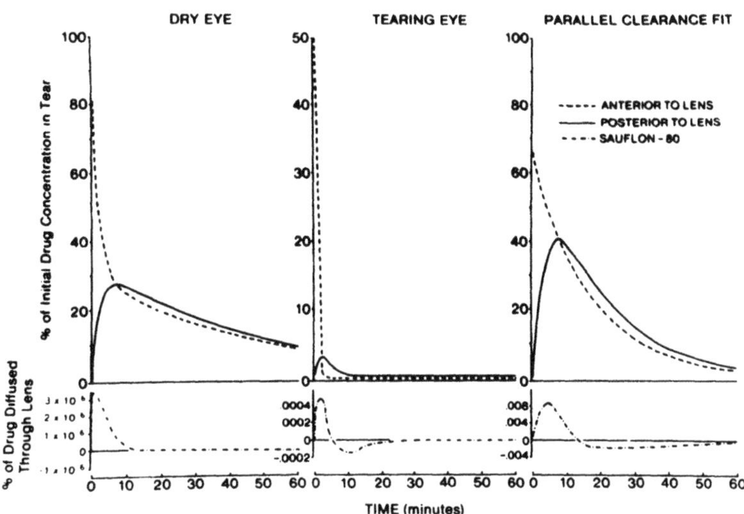

Figure 2. Kinetic model of drug distribution in the tear anterior and posterior to a 70% hydrophilic contact lens in the case of dry eye, tearing eye, and eye with parallel lens fit. The lower graphs illustrate the insignificant amount and characteristic rate of drug diffusion through the contact lens. (Cf. Mc Carey et al. 1984)

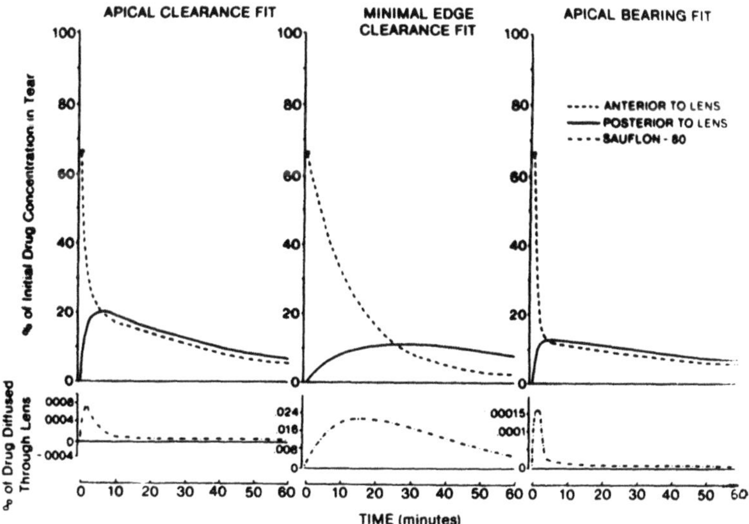

Figure 3. Kinetic model of drug distribution in th tear anterior and posterior to 70% hydrophilic contact lens that is fit on the cornea to have an apical clearance, minimal edge clearance and apical bearing. The lower graph illustrate the insignificant amount and characteristic rate of drug diffusion through the contact lens. (Cf. Mc Carey et al. 1984).

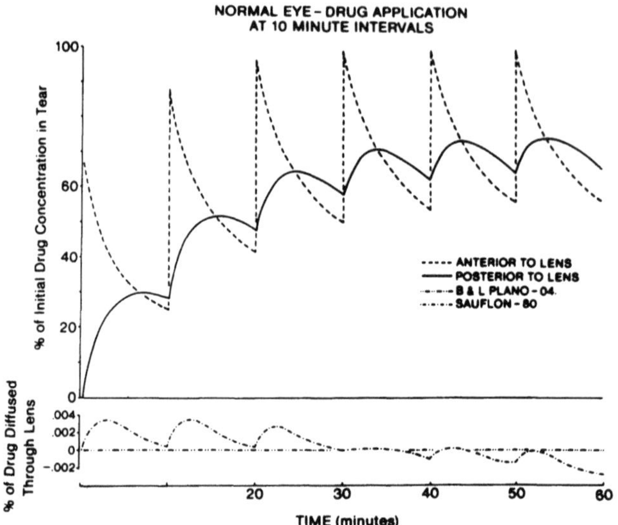

Figure 4. The upper graph illustrates the drug dilution anteriorly and posteriorly to a hydrogel lens, with a normal eye condition and with the drug reapplication at 10 minute intervals. In the lower graph, the y axis has been greatly expanded to illustrate the drug diffusion through two lenses. (Cf. Mc Carey et al , 1984).

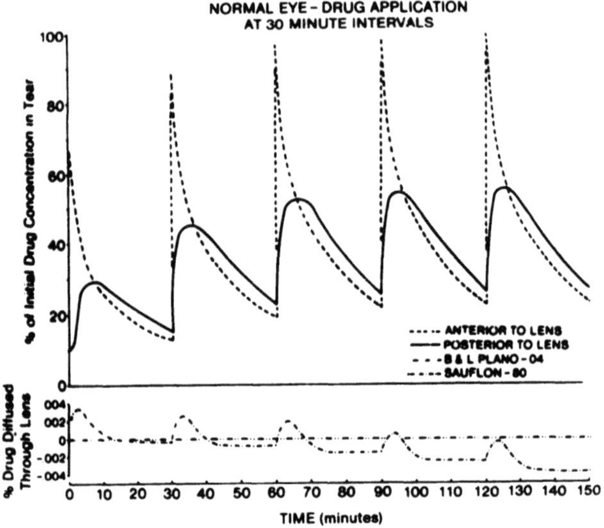

Figure 5. Same as Figure 4 except that the drug reapplications are at 30 minute intervals (Mc Carey et al. 1984).

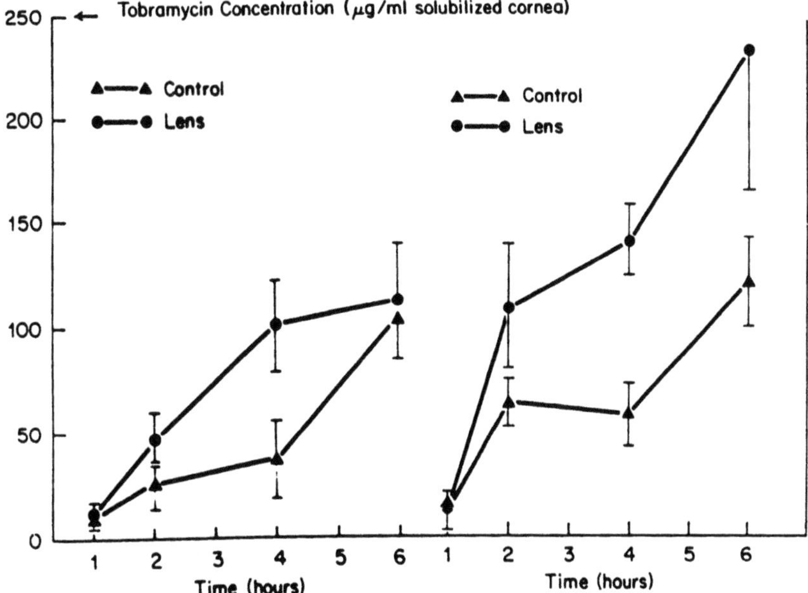

Figure 6. Corneal concentration of tobramycin in rabbits wearing low (38.6%, left) and high (71%, right) water content therapeutic soft contact lenses, following topical antibiotic administration (Matoba et al. 1985).

Presoaked contact lenses

In topical ophthalmic therapy with contact lenses, presoaked lenses are a reliable and useful drug delivery system. By means of in vitro studies the exact amount of drug adsorbed by the lens can be determined, while in vitro and in vivo studies allow a theoretical prediction of the drug release rate and of the interactions between the drug and the ocular structures. A practical knowledge of the therapeutic efficacy of medicated corneal lenses can be obtained through clinical research.

Presoaked lenses as therapeutic system are less influenced by unpredictable factors than hydrophilic lenses used in conjunction with eyedrops.

Sorensen et al. (1980) and Sorensen (1984) carried out studies on tear physiology and pathophysiology in the presence of contact lenses by means of a dynamic gamma camera and technetium. They studied the influence of contact lenses on tear flow, and the exchange of water and solutes from soft contact lenses. With their technique it was possible to make a dynamic graphical demonstration of the elimination of pertechnetate from the contact lens and from the conjunctival sac, and of its transport through the conjunctiva to the blood.

The technetium as pertechnetate was instilled on the center of a soft contact lens placed on the human eye, or used at 1/10 strength with a presoaked lens: when presoaked lenses were placed in the eye the scintigrams appeared similar to those of non-presoaked lenses.

The elimination curve in these studied seems to be monoexponential and not diphasic, as observed in normal eyes without lenses (Fig 7 and 8).

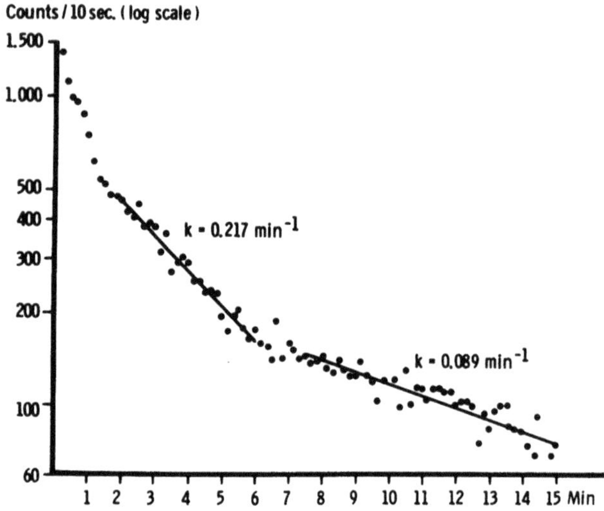

Fig. 7. Tear elimination curve in a normal eye. (Sorensen, 1984)

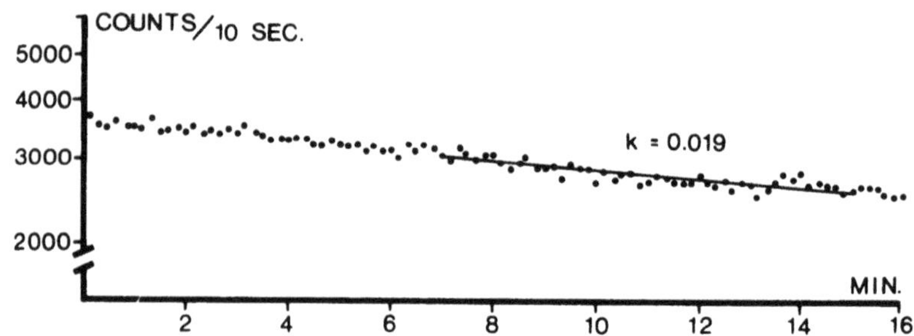

Fig.8. Tear elimination curve in a human eye fitted with a 70% hydrophilic lens. (Sorensen, 1984)

When HEMA lenses with 38% hydration were used, the elimination rate was also small (about 2% min $^{-1}$), and no significant differences were observed between the presoaked group and the group with the lens placed on the cornea during instillation of the radioisotope. After 15 min. the radioactivity had accumulated in corrispondence of the position of the soft contact lens, whereas this accumulation was not observed with hard lenses. With the latter lenses the elimination curves were diphasic as in eyes without lenses.

When soft lenses made of a different, more hydrated (75%) material were used, the pertechnetate was eliminated more slowly than from lenses containing 38% water.

The lens thickness also seems to affect the elimination

curve: with a thin lens the curve is diphasic: the radioactivity outside the lens in the conjunctival sac is relatively higher, and proportional to the total activity.

Sorensen (1984) used laboratory models for investigations with other substances, and carried out in vitro studies using lenses presoaked with pertechnetate, radioactive water ($^{3}H_2O$) and ^{14}C leucine.

In the in vitro technetium studies a good correlation with the human studies was demonstrated. The elimination was quicker with a thin lens and slower with a highly hydrated (75%) lens (Fig.9).

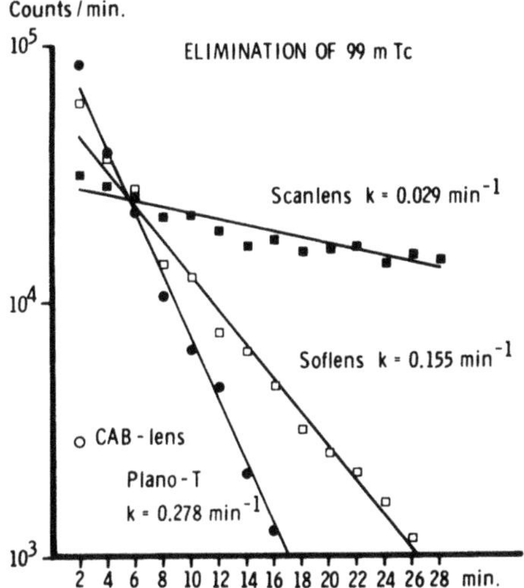

Fig. 9. Elimination of technetium from contact lenses: the radioactivity of washing solution was plotted versus time (Sorensen, 1984).

In similar studies using radioactive water it was found that water was exchanged very rapidly in the lens (Fig.10). The elimination rate was constant until the twentieth minute, then it increases suddenly.

In the study with the neutral amino acid ^{14}C leucine, no secondary elimination peak was observed. A peak (after 15 hours) was found by Hillmann (1975) in a study on the elimination of pilocarpine: some pilocarpine appeared to be bound by the lens material; water might present a similar phenomenon.

The different behavior of leucine, which was eliminated more slowly from a less hydrated lens, emphasizes the complexity of the entire problem and confirms the impossibility of theoretically predicting the diffusion rates of solutes from contact lenses under in vivo conditions.

The tracer methods applied to contact lens-wearing patients were the first to yield information on the exchange of solutes in contact lens materials in vivo. It might be possible to extend these studies by using radioactive drugs.

Hovding (1983) studied the fluid content of hydrophilic contact lenses on the eye. During wear, the fluid content of 72% hydrated lenses was about 2.5% lower than expected from in vitro

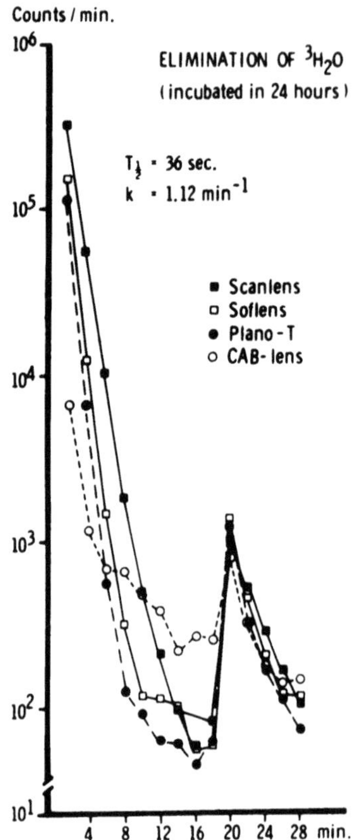

Figure 10. Elimination of radioactive water from contact lenses after a 24 hr incubation time (Sorensen 1984).

results. The difference was mainly due to the temperature susceptibility of highly hydrated lens materials.

The fluid content of hydrophilic contact lenses has been shown to increase with increasing pH of the environment. The fluid content is not significantly reduced by the mechanical pressure exerted by the eyelids.The higher the fluid content of the lens, the higher the evaporation. However, during lens wear there is normally no significant net loss of lens fluid due to evaporation.

CLINICAL EXPERIENCE

1. Use of presoaked lenses in the treatment of glaucoma.

Acute closed-angle glaucoma and chronic open-angle glaucoma are diseases in which a therapy with slow-release systems has been studied for a long time and in detail.

Since in chronic glaucoma a prolonged therapy is required,

the daily drug dosage must be minimized in order to reduce systemic side-effects without losing therapeutic efficacy.

In acute closed-angle glaucoma a high dosage of a topical drug over a short period of time is required. A drug release system produces a high drug concentration at the tissue, thus giving maximum efficacy. In classical glaucoma therapy, a large percentage of pilocarpine, introduced as solution into the conjunctival sac, is lost via the lacrimal drainage system and only 2 to 3% penetrates into the aqueous (Harris, 1968; Asseff et al., 1973).

Lerman and Raininger (1971) have shown that if pilocarpine could be administered in a slow-release form, a much smaller dose (10 to 25 times less) would be effective.

North (1971) first reported on the treatment with hydrophilic contact lenses presoaked in 4% pilocarpine of two patients with acute glaucoma . Kaufman et al (1971) showed that a soft lens combined with pilocarpine 1% drops was more effective in lowering intraocular pressure than 8% pilocarpine eyedrops alone. Podos et al. (1972) used hydrophilic lenses after a 2 min soak in pilocarpine 0.55%, and obtained a significant reduction of intraocular pressure. Their studies in vitro showed that the uptake of pilocarpine from a 0.5% solution reached a maximum after soaking for 60 min, and the release rate in vitro and in vivo approximated a half-life of 30 min, over 90% being eliminated after 4 hours of elution. Asseff et al. (1973) investigated the aqueous levels in monkey after treatment with a hydrophilic lens presoaked for 2 min in tritium-labelled 1% pilocarpine. The uptake by the bionite lens was approximately 400 µg. of pilocarpine, and the aqueous levels produced were higher than those produced by frequent eyedrops administration.

Calabria and Ciurlo (1973) used elliptic conjunctival inserts of HEMA presoaked in pilocarpine chloridrate, and found that the intraocular pressure of glaucomatous patients was lowered with a very low drug concentration. Hillman (1974) undertook a study on 25 eyes with acute closed-angle glaucoma, in order to assess the efficacy of a hydrophilic contact lens saturated with 1% pilocarpine, and to compare this method with the traditional intensive pilocarpine regimen. With presoaked contact lenses and 500 mg acetazolamide, the mean IOP decrease in two hours was 54.8%, while the mean decrease for the intensive pilocarpine (and acetazolamide) group was 49.7%.

Hillman (1974) also suggested using lenses soaked in preservative-free pilocarpine, sterilized by autoclaving in order to avoid the commonly used preservatives (benzalkonium chloride and chlorbutanol) that have a greater affinity than aqueous solutions for hydrophilic materials, and can concentrate in the lenses at levels which are toxic to the corneal epithelium. This author suggested a prolonged soak to allow an equilibration of the drug throughout the lens: with a brief soak immediately before use, pilocarpine diffuses so as to produce a gradient within the lens, the greatest concentration being at the surface, from which the drug diffuses in a shorter time and at a higher dose.

Research on the use of contact lenses in chronic glaucoma is now reduced, since better results are obtained with ocular inserts (Ocusert) which allow a continous constant-rate delivery of medications (Hales 1982). However, therapeutic contact lenses during an acute glaucomatous attack appear quite effective and remain a good form of management for this pathology.

Recent antiglaucomatous therapy is based on beta-blockers

and beta-adrenergic drugs; all these medications have various collateral systemic effects. The constant and prolonged use of these medications has emphasized thire systemic effects, together with the reduction of efficacy over time (tachyphylaxis).

Bietti et al. (1974) showed that with soft contact lenses it was possible to reduce markedly the concentration of a drug, while maintaining hypotensive effects and with no undesiderable systemic effects. This was first demonstrated with clonidine and subsequently with isoproterenol, a beta-adrenergic drug.

Isoproterenol can lower the IOP, but with systemic beta-effects on the myocardium (resulting in cardioacceleration) and on the peripheral vessels (which are dilated, resulting in decreased blood pressure).

Isoproterenol eyedrops at concentrations ranging from 1.25% to 5% cannot be instilled to reduce IOP, because the patients complain of tachycardia, arterial hypotension, anxiety and weakness when these solutions are applied.
An experimental investigation performed in rabbits indicated the possibility of administering isoproterenol at low concentrations with the aid of soft contact lenses presoaked in 0.2% isoproterenol. With a similar treatment, in 21 out of 24 glaucomatous patients a reduction in IOP ranging from 23% to 32% was observed: the therapeutic effect was obtained with a concentration (0.2%) approximately 50 times lower than that previously employed clinically (2.4%). No systemic effects, such arterial hypotension or tachycardia, were noted (Fig. 11).

However, isoproterenol is not used in glaucoma therapy and even the beta-blockers now used have important systemic effects.

In general, it is important to administer beta-blockers and antiglaucomatous drugs in low dosages if the glaucomatous patient is to be safeguarded.

2. Therapy for ocular infection with antibiotic reservoir contact lenses.

Presoaked contact lenses may be useful in the management of ocular infections and, in particular, of corneal problems.

A contact lens presoaked with antibiotic allows a more prolonged contact between the drug and the ocular tissues, a slower washout of the antibiotic by the lacrimal drainage system and, at the same time, a good protection from external agents and from lid abrasive effects.

When soft contact lenses were first used, Sedlacek (1965), Gasset and Kaufman (1970) and François and Cambie (1971) recommended lenses soaked in antibiotic solutions for the treatment of corneal ulcers.

Cerulli et al. (1981a,b, 1983) studied the pharmacokinetics of various antibiotics carried by hydrophilic contact lenses with different hydrophilic power. With the antibiotics tested, Cerulli et al. preferred less hydrophilic lenses when a prolonged treatment was required, while highly hydrophilic lenses (87%) were useful when a short-term intensive treatment was necessary.

The behaviour of different antibiotics tested with soft contact lenses varies greatly, depending on the molecular size and weight of the drug, on the temperature of the ocular surface and on the pH of the lacrimal film, as all these parameters can alter the elution of the antibiotic.

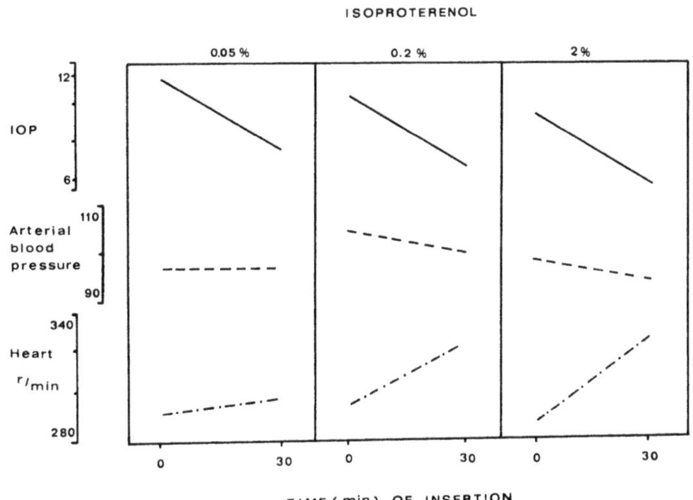

Fig. 11. Comparative effect on intraocular pressure, arterial blood pressure, and heart rate after application in rabbits of soft contact lenses presoaked respectively in 1% isoproterenol (a beta-receptor stimulating agent), 1% propranolol (a beta-blocking agent), and (on the right), in a mixture of 1% isoproterenol and 1% propanolol.

In conclusion, whenever using an antibiotic-presoaked lens it is necessary to test the lens-antibiotic system, the nature of the lens, its hydrophilic power and thickness, and the temperature and hydrogen ion concentration of the lacrimal film and of the ocular surface in different ocular pathologies. However, the data available in the literature indicate that the effect of a soft contact lens on the pharmacokinetics of topically appiled antibiotics cannot be entirely predicted.

REFERENCES

Asseff C.F., Weisman R.L., Podos S.M., Becker B. (1973). Ocular penetration of pilocarpine in primates. Am. J. Ophthalmol 75: 212-225.

Bietti G.B., Romani E., Pecori-Giraldi J. (1974). Studies on the possibility of using soft contact lenses for the administration of certain therapeutic drugs. International Medical Symposium on Soft Contact Lenses, Geneva, Nov. 1-3.

Bietti G.B., Virno M., Pecori-Giraldi J., Pellegrino N., Motolese E. (1976). Possibility of isoproterenol therapy with soft contact lenses: ocular hypotension without systemic effects. Ann: Ophthalmol 8: 819-829.

Calabria G.A., Ciurlo G. (1973). Somministrazione di farmaci mediante inserti idrofili congiuntivali. Atti 55 Congr. Soc. Oftalmol. Italiana 29: 320-326.

Cerulli L., Bagella G., Melis M., Fasulo R., Scuderi G.L. (1981b). Influenza delle variazioni della temperatura e del pH sulla farmacodinamica in vitro di antibiotici veicolati da lenti a contatto morbide. Clin. Oc. 2: 38-40.

Cerulli L., Bagella G., Fasulo R., Scuderi G.L. (1981a). Farmacodinamica di antibiotici veicolati da lenti a contatto a diverso potere idrofilo. Clin. Oc. 2: 257-260.

Cerulli L., Bagella G., Fasulo R., Martelli M. (1983). Studio sulla farmacodinamica in vitro della citosin-arabinoside veicolata da lenti a contatto morbide per il trattamento delle cheratiti erpetiche. Clin. Oc. 4: 231-234.

Ellis P.P., Matsumura M., Rendi M.A. (1985). Pilocarpine concentration in aqueous humor following single drop application. I - Effect of soft contact lenses. Curr. Eye Res. 4: 1041-1047.

François J., Cambie E. (1971). New prospectives in the treatment of corneal ulcers. T. Geneesk. 27. 1070-1074.

Gasset A., Kaufman H., (1970). Therapeutic use of hydrophilic contact lenses. Am. J. Ophthalmol. 69: 252-259.

Hales R.H. (1982). Contact lenses. A clinical approach to fitting. Baltimore, Williams & Wilkins pp. 252-259.

Harris J. (1968). In: Symposium on ocular therapy. ed. I.H. Leopold, Mosby, St. Louis, Vol. 3, p. 99.

Hillman J.S. (1974). Management of acute glaucoma with pilocarpine -soaked hydrophilic lens. Br. J. Ophthalmol. 58: 674-679.

Hillman J.S. (1975). Pilocarpine delivery by hydrophilic lens in management of acute glaucoma. Trans Ophthalmol. Soc. U.K. 95: 79-84.

Hovding G. (1983). The fluid content of hydrophilic contact lenses on the eye. Acta Ophthalmol. (Copenh). 61: 881-891.

Kaufman H.E., Uotila M.H., Gasset A.R., Wood T.O., Ellison E.D. (1971). The medical use of soft contact lenses. Trans. Am. Acad. Ophthalmol. Otolaryngol. 75: 361-373.

Lerman S., Reininger B. (1971). Simulated sustained release pilocarpine therapy and aqueous humor dynamics. Can. J. Opthalmol. 6: 14-23.

Matoba A.Y., McCulley J.P. (1985). The effect of therapeutic soft contact lenses on antibiotic delivery to the cornea. Ophthalmology 92: 97-99.

Mc Carey B.E., Wilson L.A. (1982). pH, osmolarity and temperature effects on the water content of hydrogel contact lens. Contact and Intraocular Lens Med. J. 8: 158-167.

Mc Carey B.E., Schmidt F.H., Wilkinson K.D., Baum J.P. (1984). Gentamicin diffusion across hydrogel bandage lenses and its kinetic distribution on th eye. Curr. Eye Res. 3: 977-989.

North D.P. (1971). Can. Med. Ass. J. 105: 561.

Podos S.M., Becker B., Asseff C., Hartstein J. (1972). Pilocarpine therapy with soft contact lenses. Am. J. Ophthalmol. 73: 336-341.

Sedlacek J. (1965). Possibilities of application of ophthalmic drugs with aid of gel-contact-lenses. Cs. Optalmol. 21: 509-912.

Smith S.G., Lindstrom R.L., Doughman D.G. (1982). Keratoplasty. Letter to the Editor. Ophthalmic Surg. 13: 61.

Sorensen T.B., Jensen F.T. (1980). Lacrimal pathology evaluated by dynamic lacrimal scintigraphy. Acta Ophthalmol. (Copenh) 58: 597-607.

Sorensen T.B., Jensen F.T., Marqversen J. (1980). A human and in vitro study on the exchange of water and solutes from soft contact lenses. Acta Ophthalmol. (Copenh) 58: 576-587.

Sorensen T.B. (1984). Studies on tear physiology, pathophysiology and contact lenses by means of dynamic gamma camera and technetium. Acta Ophthalmol Supp: 167: 1-53.

Waltman S., Kaufman H. (1970). Use of hydrophilic contact lenses to increase ocular penetration of topical drugs. Invest. Ophthalmol. 9. 250-255.

EFFECT OF CONTACT LENS SOLUTIONS ON THE FUNCTIONAL MORPHOLOGY OF THE CORNEA

H. Brewitt

Augenklinik der Medizinischen Hochschule Hannover
Hannover, Federal Republic of Germany

The normal corneal epithelial surface is a smooth layer with a barrier composed of tight junctions between the plasma membranes of surface cells. The surface is finely irregular, with microvilli and microplicae, and an absorbed layer of the tear film. The integrity of the precorneal film plays a key role in the optical quality of the corneal surface. Topically applied ophthalmic medications or contact lens solutions produce transient concentrations at the cornea and conjunctiva that are significantly higher than those in any other eye tissue, and may damage the tear film and the epithelial cells. Electron microscopy is particularly useful in visualization of the corneal surface reaction after application of ophthalmic solutions. This paper reports on micromorphological findings at the outer corneal surface and demonstrates that the epithelium exibits similar reactions to different noxious stimuli.

INTRODUCTION

The cornea is a functional unit which provides transparency and mechanical strength. It is convenient to consider corneal morphology and pathology on the basis of the three mayor anatomically functional components: the epithelium and its basement membrane complex, the corneal stroma and the endothelium and Descemet's membrane. The discussion of these anatomical layers is here limited to general considerations of the normal morphology necessary for an understanding and a description of reactions to topically applied drugs, in particular to contact lens solutions.

NORMAL MORPHOLOGY

Epithelium and basement membrane complex - The cornea surface has a nonkeratinized squamous epithelium of five to seven cell layers. The basal layer consist of a single layer of columnar cells that are responsible for miotic activity. Secreted by this cells in a thin, uniform basal lamina, that, together with its attendant hemidesmosomes and anchoring fibrils, makes up the attachment complexes responsible for the tight adhesion of the epithelium to the underlying Bowman's layer (Mc Tigue and Fine 1966, Hogan et al. 1971, Iwamoto et al. 1972, Brewitt and Reale 1981). Wing or polygonal cells, which form the two or three intermediate layers, contain diffusely distributed tonofilaments and a few small mitochondria. The two layers of superficial cells

Ophthalmic Drug Delivery. Biopharmaceutical, Technological and Clinical Aspects.
M.S. Saettone, G. Bucci, P. Speiser (eds.) Fidia Research Series, vol. 11, Liviana Press, Padova © 1987

are extremely flat measuring up to 40 μm in length and about 4 μm in thickness. Junctional complexes are more numerous, and very important are the tight junctions between superficial cells, which forms an important permeability and barrier. Superficial surface cells possess microvilli and microplicae of the anterior plasma membrane with fine filaments (Fig. 1a).

Another unique feature is the presence of vesicles, which contain long filaments, probably of mucus glycoprotein, that are bound to the cell membrane sorrounding the vesicle; these vesicles fuse with the cell surface, then invert and expose the mucus glycoprotein chains to the mucin of the tear film (Fig. 1b). In normal human eyes there are few vesicles, these being more frequent in rabbit corneal surface cells. The vesicles may be the first stage in the development of holes at the rabbit corneal surface (Fig. 1c). The microprojections increase tear film retention, and the filaments are probably essential factors in tear film stability (Dohlman 1971, Holly and Lemp 1977, Brewitt and Honegger 1982). The surface characteristics of these cells are best observed by scanning electron microscopy (SEM). In most species, the flat, polygonal cells possess microprojections (Blumcke and Morgenroth 1967, Leuenberger 1970, Hoffmann and Schweichel 1972/73, Pfister 1973, Honneger and Brewitt 1978). The relative density of surface microprojections accounts for the variable texture of these cells seen by SEM : "Light" cells have more microprojections then "medium-dark" and "dark" cells (Fig. 1d). This correlates well with the cell age and/or cell function. Younger and/or healthy cells have the more elaborate reticulations, whereas older and/or damaged cells have lost this plasma membrane specialisation.

Corneal stroma - The stroma consists of regular layers of collagen fibrils measuring between from 24 to 30 μm in diameter. The relatively even spacing of collagen fibrils is promoted by the glycosamminoglycans sorrounding them (Fig. 1e). There are relatively few keratocytes ; morphologically, these cells are fusiform with long cytoplastic processess. Bowan's layer, an acellular area consisting of randomly arranged collagen fibrils, is located just beneath the epithelium and the basal lamina (Hogan et al. 1971).

Endothelium and Descemet's membrane - The endothelium is a single layer of exagonal cells lining the internal surface of the cornea (Fig. 1f). Adjacent cells are extensively interdigitated and the monolayer is suited to its functions as a barrir to fluid flow. Injury of these cells may lead to edema of the epithelium and th stroma. Descemet's membrane, a true basal lamina, originates in the endothelial cells.

MORPHOLOGICAL RESPONSES OF THE CORNEA TO CONTACT LENS SOLUTIONS

The integrity of the precorneal tear film plays a key role in optical quality of the corneal surface. Topically applied ophthalmic medications produce significantly higher transient concentrations in the cornea and conjunctiva than in other ocular tissues, and may produce damage to the tear film and the epithelial cells. Contact lens solutions with their vehicles and preservatives are also present in high concentrations for a brief interval after application, or when soft contact lenses are used. These drugs may be absorbed into the lens and remain there for a longer period of time, and may damage the epithelium by disrupting the the normally resistant barrier layer. Stromal tissue may develop permanent deposits or vascularization, endothelial cells may diminish in number and function. Ocular and systemic effects of drugs on the eye are well documented (Grant 1974, Fraunfelder 1976, Burnstein 1980). In the following section are described morphological changes, particularly of the corneal epithelium, which have been demonstrated after the application of contact lens solutions. These include my findings and those reported by other authors.

Wetting or conditioner solutions are generally formulated to contain a cellulose derivative or polyvinyl alcohol. These solutions help converting a hydrophobic contact lens surface to a hydrophilic one, or are used to provide a cushion between the lens and the corneal epithelium. They are able to control tissue hydration. Topically applied PVA solutions increase the tear film breakup time and prevent epithelium cell desquamation (Fig. 2a+b) (Brewitt and Bonatz 1979). Soaking solutions are designed to prevent the drying out of the lens, to clean and to remove the protein debris from the lens surface, and to serve as a sterile medium for the lens storage. Cleansing solutions should remove dirt, oil, protein and foreign matter from the lens surface; most contain preservatives.

Benzalkonium chloride (BAC) is a quaternary ammonium compound which is usually used in concentrations of 0.01% to 0.001% in ophthalmic lens solutions. In higher concentrations, BAC can cause corneal damage in the form of desquamation of the epithelium (Fig. 2c). The epithelial cells show loss of surface microprojections and severe membrane disruption (Tonjum 1975, Pfister and Burstein 1976, Brewitt et al. 1981, Dormans and van Logten 1982, Jager et al. 1983). Delayed epithelial wound healing du to 0.01% and 0.1% BAC was shown in rabbits by Brewitt and Kunze (1981). Intracameral BAC caused irreversible edema at 0.025% to 0.05% with swelling and rupture of the endothelium (Swan 1944). The use of mercurials on the eye may cause deposits on Descemet's membrane (Fraunfelder 1976). With topical 0.002% thiomersal applications to rabbit corneas, no toxic effects were observed with scanning electron microscopy (Fig. 2d). Thiomersal 0.02% caused reduced surface microprojections and sporadic disruption of the cell membrane (Brewitt and Honegger 1982). Browne et al. (1985) found corneal irritation from soft lenses soaked in 0.01% thiomersal. Endothelial perfusion of rabbit corneas with 0.01% thiomersal produced no changes when observed by scanning or trasmission electron microscopy. At 0.01% irreversible damage with corneal swelling occured (Van Horn et al. 1977). Chlorhexidine digluconate shows low toxicity. In experiments with high doses of 0.25% to rabbits, no cell desquamation in the epithelium was found (Brewitt and Feuerhake 1980, Brewitt et al. 1981).

For a short time, contact lens cleansing and disinfecting agents acting on an oxidative basis were available. These are mainly peroxide systems. Normally, the eye does not come into contact with peroxide, a toxic oxidizing agent, that can have a corrosive effect on the eye. If cleansing and disinfection of the contact lenses is carried out incorrectly, then corneal damage is possible. We have demonstrated with the aid of scanning electron microscopy and transmission electron microscopy, that even 10 ul of 0.15% peroxide causes a little, but regularly demonstrable,

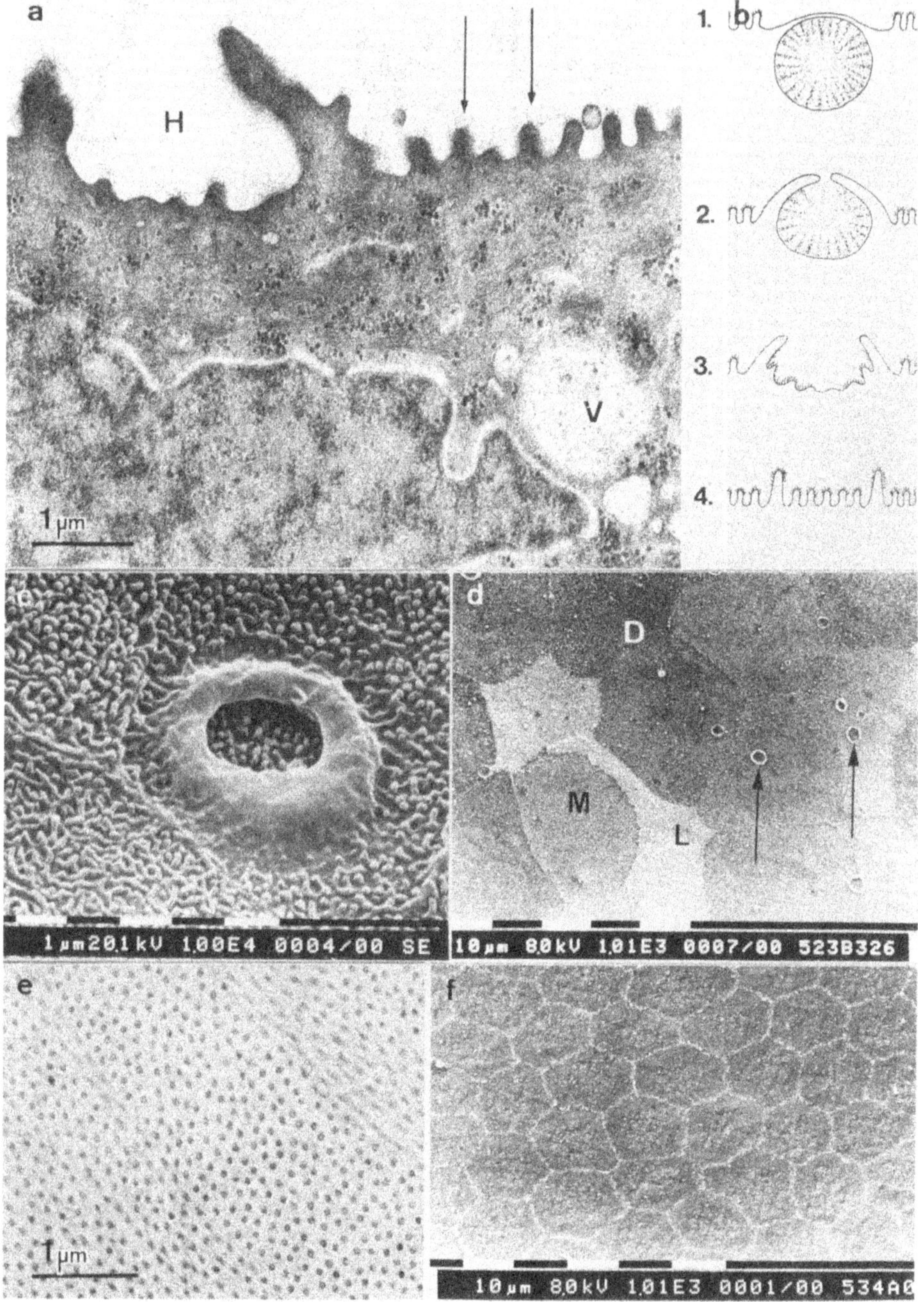

Fig. 1:a. Transmission electron micrograph (TEM) of superficial epithelial cell with numerus surface microvilli and fine

- see next page -

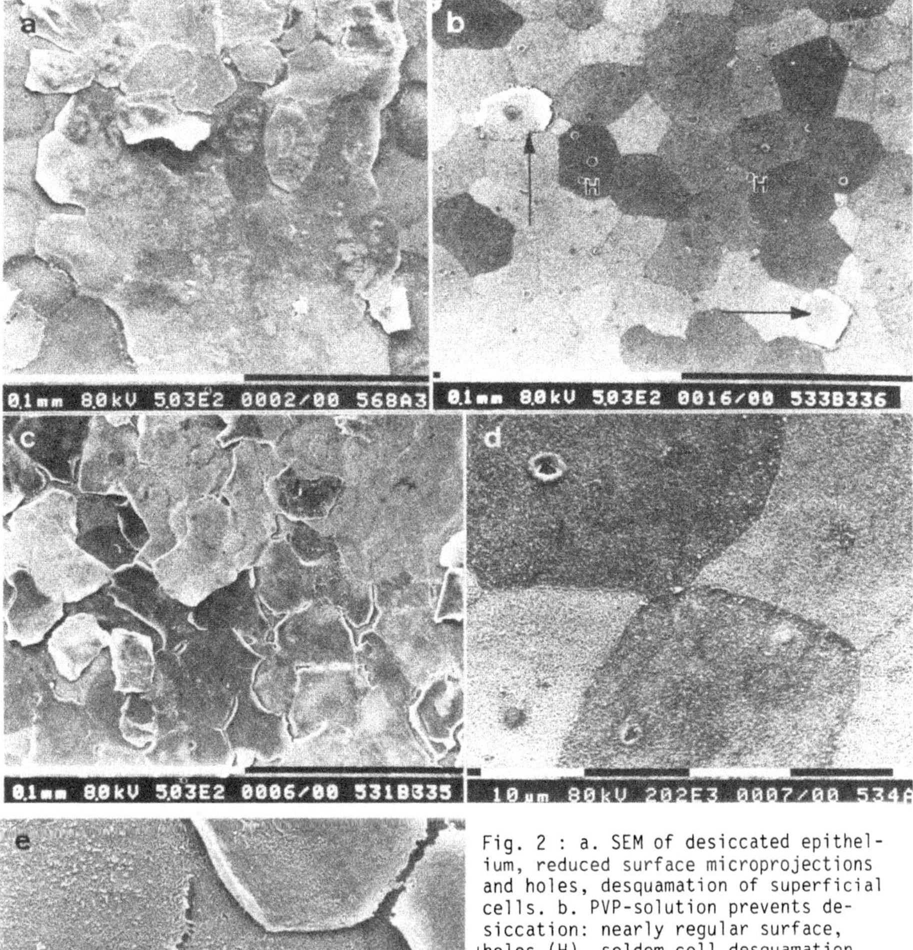

Fig. 2 : a. SEM of desiccated epithelium, reduced surface microprojections and holes, desquamation of superficial cells. b. PVP-solution prevents desiccation: nearly regular surface, holes (H), seldom cell desquamation (arrows). c. SEM of 0,1 % BAC-effects on corneal epithelium after single topical application: desquamating cells without regular surface microprojections. d. SEM of 0,002 % Thiomersal-effects on corneal surface: medium and dark cells with reduced microprojections. e. SEM of 3 % peroide-effects on corneal surface: desquamation of 2 or 3 cell layers, no regular microprojections.

---

filaments (arrows), hole (H), vesicles (V) with fine filaments. b. Model of vesicles (1) which invest to holes (2/3) and then to regular plasma membrane (4) to renew the epithelial surface. c. SEM of epithelial hole of rabbit cornea. d. SEM of epithelium of rabbit cornea: Light (L), mediumdark (M), dark (D) cells and holes (arrows). e. TEM of corneal stroma. f. SEM of endothelium of rabbit cornea: the mosaic-like pattern is normal.

cell desquamation of the rabbit cornea. Concentrations of 0.3 to 3.0% peroxide regularly cause plasma membrane defects and open cells boundaries (Fig.2e).

The application of HEMA-contact-lenses that had been stored in peroxide solutions of varying concentrations led to similar morphological reactions as those caused by the application of peroxide alone (Brewitt and Conrads 1985).

Sodium dichloroisocyanurate is another disinfectant which operates on an oxidative basis. The hypochlorite that is released is the actual oxidizing agent and is able to degrade, on the one hand, macromolecules in lens deposits and, on the other hand, compounds in micro-organism that are necessary for survival. When applied correctly, hypochlorite is labile in aqueous solution and spontaneously decomposes within 4 hours to sodium chloride, so that no micromorphological corneal damage is demonstrable. If the application is incorrect, massive cell damage can be observed in the form of pores in the plasma membrane and desquamation of the epithelial cells (Brewitt and Conrads 1986).

DISCUSSION

Most drugs have side effects which are normally recognized and usually tolerated because the side effects are offset by the therapeutic benefit received. Some preservatives, which are included in both ophthalmic drugs and normal contact solutions, have side effects that are only detectable by the subtle technique of electron microscopy in combination with animal experiments. Because of this, their use in the eye is rightly forbidden. But because of the danger of contamination they cannot be omitted from multi-dose containers. However, preservatives can bind to hydrogel contact lenses in high concentrations, so there is always a risk of local overdosage of the outer corneal surface when contact lens care agents are incorrectly used. Because of its cell toxicity, benzalkonium chloride must never be used with hydrogel lenses. Thiomersal and chlorhexidine digluconate exhibit scarcely any binding capacity with respect to the lens materials applied at present. However, overdosage of these preservatives also causes demonstrable cell reactions in the corneal epithelium.

Ophthalmic drugs or contact lens solutions, particularly when they are continually used, can alter the eye and the tear film and may cause intolerance to contact lens wear. A distinction must here be made between the systemic and the local action of the medicament. Topically applied drugs in combination with contact lenses can have an adverse effect on the corneal epithelium. An incorrect application of local anaesthetics leads to membrane effects in the epithelial cells. Antibiotics, gentamycin for example, also have a slightly damaging effect on the cell. In all cases, the precorneal tear film and the epithelial cell membran beneath it are irritated at the moment of local application (Pfister and Burstein 1976, Brewitt and Honneger 1982). Furthemore, hydrogel contact lenses can store medicaments and cause local overdosage of the cornea.
Cortisone may be mentioned as a case where undesidered effects occur in combination with contact lenses after systemic administration of medicaments. Because of a reduction in resistance, it can, amongst other things, lead to a greater propensity towards infection of the very sensitive bradytrophic cornea.

The main area threatened by local administration of ophthalmics is the corneal epithelium with its precorneal film. Medicament-dependent changes to this tissue layer exibit a similar micromorphological picture as does destruction of the precorneal film (Pfister and Burnstein 1976, Brewitt and Bonatz 1979, Brewitt et al. 1979, Brewitt and Honegger 1982). Experimental exposure to air leads to a reduction in the microvilli and microplicae and a loss of the fine filaments. Holes are not usually found in dessicated cells. This confirms the hypotesis that the vesicles pushed to the surface take a part in the formation of the outer plasma membrane with their microfilaments.

Dessiccated cells, where the precorneal film is interrupted, react with the loss of microprocesses and holes. The loss of holes is characteristic of the epithelial reaction after the administration of drugs. The various noxae cause a uniform type of cell damage, which should probably be regarded as the expression of damage to the precorneal film.

REFERENCES

Blumcke S., Morgenroth K. (1967). The Stereo Ultrastructure of the External and Internal Surface of the Cornea. J. Ultrastruct. Res. 18:502-518

Brewitt H., Bonatz E. (1979). Experimentelle Untersuchungen uber die Austrocknung des Hornhautepithels. Contactologia 1: 26-37.

Brewitt H., Honegger H., Konitz H. (1979). Rasterelektronenmikroskopische Untersuchungen uber die Austrockung des Hornhautepithels un die Wirkung von Tranenersatzflussigkeiten. Klin. Mbl. Augenheilkd. 175: 521-529.

Brewitt H., Feuerhake C. (1980). Der Einfluss von Desinfektionslosungen fur HEMA-Kontactlinsen auf das Hornhautepithel - Eine rasterelektronenmikroskopische Untersuchung. Contactologia 2: 262-272.

Brewitt H., Kunze G. (1981). Zum Einfluss von Benzalkoniumchlorid auf die Wundheilung der Hornhaut. Contactologia 4: 183-190

Brewitt H., Kunze G., Konitz H. (1981). Zytotoxizitat von Konservierungsstoffen in Augenmedikamentem. Eine rasterelktronenmikroskopische Untersuchung an der Kaninchencornea. Beitr. elektronenmikroscop. Direktabb. Oberfl. 14: 543-548.

Brewitt H., Reale E. (1981). The basement membrane complex of the human corneal epithelium. Albrecht von Graefes Arch. Klin. Ophthalmol. 215: 223-231.

Brewitt H., Honegger H. (1982) . Morphologische Befunde des Hornhautepithels bei Storung des praecorneal Filmes und nach Applikation von Augenmedikamenten. Eine raster - und trasmissionselektronenmicroskopische Untersuchung. In: Marquardt R (ed): Chronische Conjunctivitis - Trockenes Auge. Springer, Vienna pp 35-57 .

Brewitt H., Conrads S. (1985). Morphologische Beunde der Hornhaut unter dem Einfluss von Peroxiol (H2O2). Contactologia 7: 116-125.

Brewitt H., Conrads S. (1986). Erfahrungen mit dem Kontaktlinsen-Desinfection und Reinigungsmittel Natriumdichlorisocyanurat. Z. prakt. Augenheilk. 7: 67-70.

Browne R.K., Anderson A.N., Charvez B.W., Azzarello R.J. (1985). Ophthalmic response to chlorhexidine digluconate in rabbits. Toxicol. Appl. Pharmacol. 32: 621-627.

Burnstein N.L. (1980). Corneal cytotoxicity of topically applied drugs, vehicles and preservatives. Surv. Ophthalmol. 25: 15-30.

Dohlman C.H. (1971). The function of the corneal epithelium in health and disease. Invest. Ophthalmol. 10: 383-407.

Dormans J.A.M., van Lotgen M.J. (1982). The effects of ophthalmic preservatives on corneal epithelium of the rabbit: a scanning microscopial study. Toxicol. Appl. Pharmacol. 62: 251-261.

Fraunfelder F.T. (1976). Drug-induced ocular side effects and drug interactions. Lea & Febiger, Philadelphia.

Grant W.M. (1974). Toxicology of the eye. Thomas, Springfield.

Hoffmann F., Schweichel J.U. (1972/73). The microvilli structure of the corneal epithelium of the rabbit in relation to cell function. A trasmission and scanning electron microscopy study. Ophthal. Res. 4: 175-184.

Hogan M.J., Alvarado J.A., Weddell J.E. (1971). Histology of the human eye. An atlas and textbook. Saunders, Philadelphia Londopn Toronto.

Holly F.J., Lemp M.A. (1977). Tear physiology and dry eyes. Surv. Ophthalmol. 22: 69-87.

Honegger H., Brewitt H. (1978). Das normale Hornhaut - und Bindehautepithel im Rasterelektronenmikroskopischen Bild. Ber. Dtsch. Ophthalmol. Ges. 75: 646-648.

Iwamoto T., DeVoe A.G., Farris R.L. (1972). Electron microscopy in cases of marginal degeneration of the cornea. Invest. Ophthalmol. 11: 241-257.

Jager M., Brewitt H., Rieger S., Konitz H. (1983). Untersuchungen zur Morphologie des Hornhautepithels nach Lagzeitanwendund von Konservierungsstoffen. Beitr. elektronenmikroskop. Direkttabb. Oberfl. 16: 459-464.

Leuenberger P.M. (1970) Die Stereo-Ultrastruktur der Cornealoberflache bei der Ratte. Albrecht von Graefes Arch. Klin. Ophthalmol. 180: 182-192.

Mc Tigue J.W., Fine B.S. (1966). The basement membrane of corneal epithelium. In:Uyeda R (ed): Electron microscopy. Maruzen Co Ltd, Tokyo; pp. 775-776.

Pfister R.R. (1973). The normal surface of corneal epithelium: A scanning electron microscopy study. Invest. Ophthalmol. 12: 654-668.

Pfister R.R., Burnstein N.L. (1976). The effects of ophthalmic drugs, vehicles, and preservatives on corneal epithelium: a scanning electron microscope study. Invest. Ophthalmol. 15: 246-259.

Swan K.C. (1944). Reactivity of the ocular tissue to wetting agents. Am. J. Ophthamol. 27: 1118-1122.

Tonjum A.M. (1975). Effects of benzalkonium chloride upon the corneal epithelium studied by scanning electron microscopy. Acta Ophthal. 53: 358-366.

Van Horn D.L., Edelhauser H.F., Prodanovich G., Eiferman R., Pederson H.J. (1977). Effect of the ophthalmic preservative thimerosal on rabbit and human corneal epithelium. Invest. Ophthalmol. 16: 273-280.

STRUCTURE, COMPOSITION AND PHYSIOPATHOLOGY OF THE LACRIMAL FILM

S. Liotet and O. Kogbe

Centre National d'Ophtalmologie des Quinze-Vingts
28, Rue de Charenton, 75012 Paris, France

1) STRUCTURE OF THE LACRIMAL FILM

The formation of the lacrimal film is the result of a precarious equilibrium, contributed to by many anatomical, physiological, mechanical and physical factors. As the subject is so vast, we will deal briefly with what is already well known, and will then focus on the more recent advances, and on the clinical and pharmacological applications of our present knowledge of the lacrimal film.

The lacrimal film breaks up and is reformed at each blink. Blinking gives an effect which Jones (1) labelled "lacrimal pump".

At the same time, with the eyelid movement, a lipid layer originating in the Meibomian glands is deposited on the lacrimal film surface, and a film of mucus is spread on the epithelial surface.

Between two consecutive blinks, the lacrimal film spreads out in a particular fashion over the ocular surface. Wright (2), using fine carbon particles, demonstrated the presence of two zones: an active zone, in which secreted tears move around in correspondence of the lacrimal river along the lids, and from which tears are drained, and a static zone, devoid of currents, corresponding to the precorneal area. The latter zone is actually subject to some important physical modifications, due to increased evaporation.

The lacrimal film has a thickness of about 7 μ, and is made up of:

1) an innermost layer, which, according to Lemp et al. (3) is formed of mucus originating from the goblet cells and from the glands of Henle;

2) a middle aqueous layer, which is the most important, and is secreted by the main lacrimal glands and those of Wolfring and Krause;

3) an outermost lipid layer, which maintains the lacrimal film and minimizes evaporation, and is essentially derived from the secretion of the Meibomian glands.

The normal volume of the lacrimal film, 5 to 9 μl, can be reduced after local anaesthesia. The flow, which is usually about 1 μl/min, can be increased by local irritants, and reduced following local anaesthesia. This, according to Jones (1), proves that there is a basal secretion and a reflex secretion, a theory that is contested by other authors.

How the lacrimal film clings to the corneo-conjunctival surface.

The conjunctival surface is normally hydrophobic. The fixation of the lacrimal film onto this surface depends mainly

Ophthalmic Drug Delivery. Biopharmaceutical, Technological and Clinical Aspects.
M.S. Saettone, G. Bucci, P. Speiser (eds.) Fidia Research Series, vol. 11, Liviana Press, Padova

upon a phenomenon of wettability. According to Holly and Lemp (4), the conjunctival mucus in indispensable in lowering surface tension, and is the wetting agent which allows the lacrimal film to spread over the corneo-conjunctival surface. Although we agree that a wetting agent is necessary, we don't believe that this agent is the conjunctival mucus, as many observations contradict this theory, the main ones being the following:
-the absence of goblet cells in the cornea;
-human conjunctival mucus is a very high molecular weight polymer, and forms a partially insoluble gel whose presence can be demonstrated by coloration or by using carbon particles;
-certain mammals (particularly rodents) do not blink or rarely do so, yet their lacrimal film is normal.

For the above reasons, we suggest that the wetting agent of the ocular surface is glycocalix, a mucoprotein which forms a cell-coat on the epithelium, and is produced by all the epithelial cells of the cornea and conjunctiva. Microscopic observations of epithelial cells indeed reveal the formation of vesicles containing a branched-out substance, which is discharged on the surface of the cells, where it is fixed onto microvilli, probably on specific sites. The formation of the preocular lacrimal film, in our opinion, is not due to mucus but to glycocalix which ensures the anchorage of the lacrimal film to the epithelium, thus securing its stability.

The roles of the lacrimal film

The lacrimal film prevents dryness of the epithelial cells by maintaining the proper humidification. Furthermore, a) it ensures a mechanical protection of the cornea and conjunctiva against variations of temperature, wind, dust and other foreign bodies; b) it ensures an extremely important immune protection through very complex specific and non-specific immunological systems; c) it plays a cleaning-up role by means of mucus, which intercepts solid particles and eliminates them from the ocular surface; d) it plays a metabolic role, particularly for the nutrition of the epithelial cells of the cornea which are avascular, as it is rich in enzymes of the energy metabolism, lysosomial enzymes and other nutritional substances; e) it plays an optical role by polishing the corneal surface, and f) it plays a lubricating role, by facilitating the sliding of the eyelids over the corneo-conjunctival surface.

The regulation of tear secretion

There is a well-known regulation of reflex tearing by the nervous system, but probably also a humoral regulation, which might be under the influence of prolactin.

The regulation of mucus secretion may, according to Franklin and Bang (5), be influenced by a humoral factor, which they name the muco-stimulating factor. The density of the goblet cells could also depend on the epithelial concentration of cyclic A.M.P. Vitamin A plays an important part in the goblet cell concentration.

The lipid regulation could be mechanical, by the contraction of the eyelids as it occurs during weeping. There might also be a humoral regulation, since androgens increase this secretion while oestrogens decrease it.

Many pharmacological substances can modify tear secretion either by acting on the nervous regulation, or by blocking the spheno-palatine ganglion: anaesthetics have this effect.

2) COMPOSITION OF THE LACRIMAL FILM

We here outline the main points essential to pharmacologists and clinicians.

The main physical characteristics of the lacrimal film are the following:

- the pH value, once estimated as 7.6 to 7.8, has now been found to be more variable. Recent studies with micro-electrodes show that with closed lids the pH becomes acid, falling to 6.5, while with open lids the pH rises progressively, stabilising in about 50 seconds at 9.3. Therefore, at each blink the pH change is in the order of 1.5 to 2 units.

The osmolarity is also an important physical factor. According to Gilbard et al. (6) its value is 304 ± 10 mOsm/l in normal subjects.

In tears, there are many substances with concentrations approaching those in serum while other ones are present at much lower concentrations: glucose is 15 times less concentrated in tears than in serum.

The tear proteins

The concentration of the tear proteins ranges from 4 to 10 g/l. Two-dimensional separation methods have revealed at least 60 different tear proteins, which can be classified into the following 3 groups:

a) proteins synthesized from the lacrimal glands;
b) proteins filtering from the vascular sector and crossing the hemolacrimal barrier;
c) proteins sinthesized locally, especially in the lymphoid tissue of the conjunctival epithelium.

a) The proteins synthesized in the lacrimal gland form the bulk of tear proteins, representing about 99% of total tear proteins. The main proteins of this group are:

- the fast migrating proteins, a group of low molecular weight proteins which migrate faster than albumin, and whose role is not yet known.
- the protein G.

Fast migrating proteins and protein G are specific tear proteins.

- Proteins from the non-specific immune system, which are common to all secretions, i.e.:
  - lysozyme, which is a muramidase attacking the wall of Gram+ bacteria;
  - lactoferrin, a major tear protein, which is an iron-binding protein, and a true antibiotic;
  - the secretory immunoglobulin A, which is part of the specific immune defence system of the mucosa.

b) Proteins filtering from the vascular sector through the hemolacrimal barrier.

The lacrimal film can be considered a liquid collection in which the concentration of serum proteins varies very little, because there is an equilibrium between the concentration of these proteins in serum and in tears.

The hemolacrimal barrier is very tight, thus very few

serum proteins filter into tears: only about 1% of the total. The following proteins have been reported:

-albumin, which is the most important, and whose concentration is used to determine the permeability of the hemo-lacrimal barrier;

-immunoglobulins, present in very low concentrations;

-antiproteases like alpha 1 antitrypsin, alpha 1 antichymotrypsin, alpha 2 macroglobulin;

-complement proteins, C3 proconvertase, C3;

-other proteins, such as haptoglobin, Zn alpha 2 glycoprotein and transferrin.

c) Proteins synthesized in the epithelium.

In normal subjects this synthesis is very low, but it can be extremely important in infectious pathology or even during an allergic reaction.

Tears are extremely rich in enzymes whose concentrations can attain levels 15 to 100 fold those found in serum. Pratically all the metabolic enzymes, lysosomal enzymes and others such as the angiotensinogen conversion enzyme can be found in tears. Tears also contain some hormones, prolactin, T3, T4, and insulin having been found.

The analysis of lacrimal proteins in current and clinical practice can be carried out in two ways:

-electrophoresis, which reflects the functional activity of the lacrimal gland, as 3 main peaks correspond to the major tears proteins. These, from the anode to the cathode, are:

- the fast migrating proteins
- lactoferrin
- lysozime, which migrates to the cathode.

Any alteration in the lacrimal gland shows up in elctrophoresis by a decrease in one or more of these fractions.

- The permeability of the hemolacrimal barrier can be studied through the assay of tear albumin and tear IgG, and may reveal, for example, a subclinical inflammation. Only a very simple calculation is needed to ascertain whether there is a local synthesis of IgG.

The same principle can be used to reveal a local synthesis of immunoglobulin E during allergic reactions.

Mucus

Mucus is made up of mucoproteins, some of which are secreted by the goblet cells, while glycocalix is secreted by the epithelial cells.

The structure of mucus allows easy absorption and retention of water. The coloration of mucus shows that it is present on the ocular surface as threads or as a meshwork which is capable of trapping foreign bodies. Apart from this role, the others are:

-water reservoir;

-lubricant; which facilitates the sliding of the eyelids on the ocular surface.

The lipid layer

In subjects with a normal tear film there is a great variation in the proportions of the different lipids present in the lipid layer.

The role of this layer is to prevent the evaporation of the aqueous layer and to stabilise the tear film.

3) PHYSIOPATHOLOGY OF THE LACRIMAL FILM

Anomalies affecting the different layers of the lacrimal film can be either quantitative or qualitative.

1) Anomalies of the mucus layer.

There could be:

- a hypersecretion of conjunctival mucus, as it is commonly seen in inflammatory reactions of different origin, and also in contact lens wearers.

Some affections leading to destruction or depletion of the goblet cells result in an important diminution or even in a disappearance of mucus. Vitamin A deficiency, and all diseases resulting in conjunctival scarring with goblet cell destruction are essentially responsible for this condition. Qualitative anomalies in mucus have never been encountered.

2) Anomalies of aqueous layer.

The quantitative modifications could be due to:

- inflammation, with an increase in the permeability of the hemolacrimal barrier. As a consequence, the concentration of proteins from serum, which normally should be around 1%, increases, thus raising the overall tear protein concentration to 20-30 g/l or even more. Serum proteins could thus become the major proteins in the tears. A diagnosis is easily made make by albumin and IgG assay.

- local synthesis of specific immunoglobulins, following stimulation by an antigen of whatever origin (viral, bacterial, fungal or even allergic).

Others anomalies affecting the tear protein composition are due to disfunction of the lacrimal gland. Two such affections are:

- keratoconjunctivitis sicca, in which tissue alteration results in a failure to synthesize lacrimal proteins in the lacrimal gland. This is easily detected by tear electrophoresis, which shows a diminution or disappearance of one or more proteins normally synthesized by the lacrimal gland.

- the other is a syndrome, demonstrated several years ago by us, in which specific antibacterial proteins disappear and new proteins are synthesized. This syndrome, which is generally temporary, was discovered in contact lens wearers whose hydrophilic lenses clog rapidly. We described two types: type I, in which all normal tear proteins are absent, and are replaced by new proteins, and type II which is intermediate between type I and the normal type.

3) Anomalies of the lipid layer.

This layer can be absent in rare cases of congenital absence of Meibomian glands.

The lipids can be altered during infections, e.g. by Staphylococcus, which produces a lipase, or for environmental reasons, as it occurs for example to dry cleaners working with organic solvents.

The lipid layer could also be contaminated by hydrocarbons present in the environment, e.g. from exhaust fumes of cars, and by cutaneous sebum, which quickly destroys the lipid layer as it happens in some dermatoses like acne rosacea.

4) Formation of dry spots and consequent cellular lesions.

a) Holly hypothesis - According to Holly and Lemp (4), the formation of dry spots is due to contamination of the mucus layer by fats when the lacrimal film becomes very thin. This contamination occurs easily because there is a gradient of tension at the interior of the film and irregularities at the corneo-conjunctival surface. The contaminated mucus becomes hydrophobic and a dry spot appears in the contaminated zone which results in epithelial suffering. According to these authors, the goblet cells play a very important role, and a decrease in goblet cell count would be the initial cause of tear film instability. This decrease occurs in keratoconjunctivitis sicca and in many other infections.

b) Our hypotesis - This is based on the assumption that the stability of the lacrimal film is not due to mucus from the goblet cells but to glycocalix from the epithelial cells. In our opinion, all causes of dryness eventually result in epithelial suffering.

Where there are anomalies of the lipid layer, as e.g. in lagophthalmos, inocclusion of the eyelids, exophthalmos, etc., an increased evaporation will follow, resulting in hyperosmolarity of tears. As shown by Gilbard et al. (6), this hyperosmolarity is toxic to the epithelial cells, and leads to epithelial suffering and to destruction of the goblet cells. Thus, the disappearance of the goblet cells is the result, not the cause of ocular dryness.

Vitamin A deficiency, which disturbs epithelial cellular differentiation, will result in the same anomaly of epithelial cells. Poor tear quality results in epithelial undernourishment and suffering. From the moment the epithelial cell suffers, there is a decrease in or an arrest of glycocalix synthesis resulting in a corneal hydrophobia.

When the cornea is hydrophobic, the lacrimal film is ruptured with conseguent epithelial suffering. This vicious circle must be interrupted by drug treatment if the condition is to be healed.

Likewise, all bullous dermatoses and all scarring of the conjunctiva which destroy goblet cells also destroy epithelial cells, and result in formation of scarred tissues, which are devoid of secretory vesicles for the production of glycocalix which stabilizes the tear film.

CONCLUSION

The formation and stability of the lacrimal film is very precarious. Local therapy should strive to preserve the existing fragile equilibrium, to prevent injury to the corneo-conjunctival surface and to respect tear physiology.

It should always be borne in mind that glycocalix is synthesized by epithelial cells, as we have repeatedly observed signs of epithelial suffering in all the pathologies we have studied by conjunctival imprint cytology.

This should result in a new attitude towards corneo-conjunctival conditions, which should be managed in a special way, with a particular awareness of the need to restore the normal corneo-conjunctival functions.

REFERENCES

1) Jones, L.T. The lacrimal secretory system and its treatment. Am. J. Ophthalmol, 62, 47-60 (1966).

2) Wright, P. Normal tear production and drainage. Trans. Ophthalmol. Soc. 104, 351-354 (1985).

3) Lemp, M.A., Holly, F.J., Iwata, S. and Dohlman, C.H. The precorneal tear film I. Factors in spreading and maintaining a continuous tear film over the corneal surface. Arch. Ophthalmol. 83, 89-94 (1970).

4) Holly, F.J. and Lemp, M.A. Wettability and wetting of corneal epithelium. Exp. Eye Res. 11, 239-250 (1971).

5) Franklin, M. and Bang, B.C., Mucus-stimulating factors in tears. J. Invest. Ophthalmol. 19, 430-432 (1980).

6) Gilbard, J.P., Carter, J.B., Verges, C., Refojo, M.F. et al. Effect of hyperosmolarity on ocular surface epithelium in vivo. Proc. VIIth Congr. Eur. Soc. Ophthalmol., Helsinki, 21-25 May 1984, p. 354-358.

NANOPARTICLES AND LIPOSOMES IN OPHTHALMIC DRUG DELIVERY

J. Kreuter

Institut für Pharmazeutische Technologie
Johann Wolfgang Goethe Universität, 6000 Frankfurt/Main, West Germany

The drainage and ocular distribution of nanoparticles and liposomes was investigated using the labelling of the nanoparticle polymer with ^{14}C and the binding of a tracer, ^{111}In-oxine, on to the particles and to the liposomes. The longest precorneal half-life was observed with positively charged liposomes yielding an about 3-fold increase in comparison to a simple solution. The half-life in the inner canthus was prolonged from 5 min to about 20 min. In the inner canthus, nanoparticles had the longest half-life. About 1 % of the initial nanoparticle dose adhered to the corneal and conjunctival surfaces for over 6 hours. While a lower ophthalmic absorption of the lipophilic drug progesterone was observed, a 1.4-fold higher efficacy of the more hydrophilic drug pilocarpine was obtained after binding to nanoparticles as determined by miosis measurements.

INTRODUCTION

The topical application of a drug to the eye in a conventional solution results in extensive drug loss. Therefore, only a small amount (1 - 3 %) actually penetrates the cornea and reaches intraocular tissues, while the majority of the drug is rapidly eliminated from the eye via lacrimal drainage (Wood et al., 1985; Patton and Robinson, 1976; Lee and Robinson, 1979). As a consequence, most drug becomes systemicly absorbed via the nose or via the gut possibly leading to side-effects.

Ointments and, especially drug inserts, can effectively prolong the absorption times (Sieg and Robinson, 1979; Macoul and Pavan-Langston, 1975). However, both systems can mechanically obscure the vision significantly or, in the case of the inserts, many patients, especially the elderly, have problems with the insertion and removal of these inserts.

For this reason, biodegradable polycyanoacrylate nanoparticles as ocular delivery systems were evaluated and compared to liposomes. Polycyanoacrylates have been successfully used in surgery as tissue adhesives for almost 20 years. Nanoparticles are colloidal particles, ranging in size from 10 to 1000 nm, in which drug may be entrapped, encapsulated, and/or adsorbed. In view of the fact that previous work has shown a relationship between particle size and precorneal retention (J.W. Sieg, personal communication), that polyalkyl-2-cyanoacrylates and related polymers have been shown to be bioadhesive, and that bioadhesive polymers have potential

Ophthalmic Drug Delivery. Biopharmaceutical, Technological and Clinical Aspects.
M.S. Saettone, G. Bucci, P. Speiser (eds.) Fidia Research Series, vol. 11, Liviana Press, Padova © 1987

to improve drug delivery in general, nanoparticles may be a useful dosage form for ocular drug delivery.

The drainage and ocular distribution of nanoparticles and degradation products was investigated using the labelling of the nanoparticle polymer with ^{14}C (Wood et al., 1985) and the binding of a tracer, ^{111}In-oxine, on to the particles.

OCULAR DISPOSITION OF ^{14}C-LABELLED NANOPARTICLES

In-vitro degradation of the nanoparticles in tears occurred at a relatively rapid rate for the first hour with approximately 19 % degradation followed by a general levelling off over the next 5 h. The decrease in degradation rate may be caused by a decrease in enzyme activity during the experiment.

The half life of clearance from the tear film is approximately 15 to 20 min versus less than 2 min with solutions (Wood et al., 1985; Fig. 1). Approximately 0.1 % of the initial amount of nanoparticles

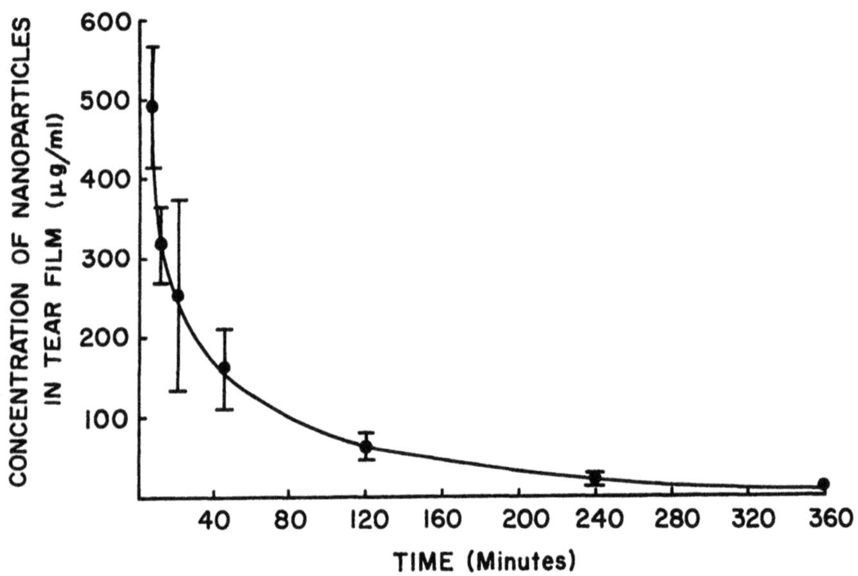

Figure 1
Concentration versus Time Profile of Nanoparticles in the Tear Film

was found to be associated with the cornea for 6 hours. This points to bioadhesive properties of these particles. More than 0.6 % was found to be associated with the conjunctiva for the same time.

Therefore approximately 1 % of the initial nanoparticles adheres to cornea and conjunctiva.

Besides bioadhesion, uptake by endocytoticly active tissue may be an explanation of this long association of the nanoparticle with the conjunctiva, of course not the cornea. Nevertheless, bioadhesion seems to be more likely. The structural features of the polymer i.e. charge density and hydrophobicity, are similar to those of polymers that have been previously shown to possess bioadhesive properties.

One of the existing theories regarding the mechanism of bioadhesion is that bioadhesive polymer adheres at the mucin-epithelial surface of cells. To determine the effect of mucin on the interaction between the nanoparticles and conjunctival and corneal tissue, animals were predosed with N-acetyl-L-cysteine, a known mucolytic agent before instilling the nanoparticle suspension. There was no significant difference between treatments for the cornea and aqueous humor suggesting that the nanoparticles are able to adhere directly to corneal tissue (Wood et al., 1985). The results also indicated that the mucin layer does not appear to represent a barrier to permeation of the cornea by degradative products of the polymer. However, there was a significantly higher conjunctival concentration of nanoparticles when the eye was treated with the mucolytic agent. Upon treatment with the mucolytic agent, it was observed that quantities of mucin collected in the cul-de-sac forming a gel-like substance. It is probable that nanoparticles became entrapped in this substance, and this may account for the higher conjunctival concentration with N-acetyl-L-cysteine treatment.

For drug solutions applied topically to the eye, it has been shown that only the first 5 min are important for corneal absorption. After 5 min, due to rapid loss of drug from the tear film, negligible amounts of drug are absorbed by the cornea. Therefore, if about 1 % of the nanoparticle dose is retained in the precorneal area by adhesion to the cornea and conjunctival tissue, contact time between the dosage form and the absorbing tissue is increased (Wood et al., 1985).

Very low radioactivity was found in the aqueous humor with a peak level after 1 h (Wood et al., 1985). Intact nanoparticles are very likely unable to permeate the cornea and enter the anterior segment. Since it is known that the nanoparticles biodegrade upon instillation into the tear film, the measured chemical in the aqueous humor is probably not nanoparticles but rather a degradation product.

ELIMINATION KINETICS OF ^{111}In-LABELLED NANOPARTICLES

In another experiment, the particles were labelled with ^{111}In-oxine after polymerization at a neutral pH. Over 98 % of the label was thus associated with the nanoparticles. The use of the ^{111}In-oxine as the labelling agent allowed the use of a gamma-camera equiped with a pinhole collimator. Thus the kinetics of the nanoparticle clearance could be studied without sacrifice of the animal. This clearance was compared to liposomes.

The clearance of solutions as well as of both types of colloidal carriers from the cornea is much faster than from the inner canthus. However, ocular absorption is possible from both areas, but probably not from the lacrimal duct.

The solutions had clearance half lifes of 1.3 min for the cornea and 5 min for the inner canthus. The largest corneal half life of 3.7 min was observed with positive small unilamellar vesicles. Probably due to their positive charge, these vesicles adhere longer to the negatively charged corneal surface. Nanoparticles had a corneal half life of 2.2 min and the longest inner canthus half life of 17.3 min. This value corresponds well to the half life calculated by the tear radioactivity elimination with ^{14}C-labelled nanoparticles.

OCULAR DISPOSITION OF PROGESTERONE INCORPORATED INTO NANOPARTICLES

In another experiment, the ocular distribution kinetics of a very lipophilic model compound - ^{3}H-progesterone - was tested (Li et al., 1986). This drug is very water insoluble. As a result, over 99 % of the progesterone in a 2 x 10^{-5} molar preparation was sorbed to the nanoparticles. Since the nanoparticles represented only 1 % of the total volume, under the assumption of drug uptake by partitioning, a water/nanoparticle partition coefficient of 1/10000 would result. The assumption of a linear partitioning coefficient seems to be valid, because this was observed with similar systems.

The progesterone concentrations obtained with nanoparticles were about 4 times lower than those obtained with the solution. Similar results were obtained in the conjunctiva and in the cornea. Probably due to the high affinity of the drug to the particles, the contact time in the eye is still too short to allow for a sufficient release and ocular absorption of this drug.

Although the nanoparticle payload of this drug may be enhanced considerably due to the high partitioning coefficient, which in turn may enhance the amount available for ocular absorption, it has to be taken into consideration that the majority of the drug still may not be absorbed in the eye but rather later in the body which then could lead to unwanted systemic effects.

For this reason, a more hydrophilic drug, pilocarpine, in the form of its nitrate and its hydrochloride salt was evaluated for an optimization of ocular drug delivery by binding to nanoparticles (Harmia et al., 1986 a,b,c).

PILOCARPINE NANOPARTICLES

Two different methods of drug loading of pilocarpine onto nanoparticles were studied: Firstly, binding by sorption to the particles after their polymerization and secondly, the incorporation by polymerization in presence of the drug. Particles of a size around 400 nm were produced.

The most suitable polymer material for the pilocarpine adsorption was polybutylcyanoacrylate. Electrolytes enhanced the adsorption of pilocarpine. The most optimal electrolyte tested was sodium sulfate. Surfactants also somewhat increased the adsorption of pilocarpine onto the nanoparticles. The sorption enhancing effect increased with increasing carbon side-chain length. Polysorbate 80 had a better effect than polysorbate 20. However, the best results were obtained with Brij 35 and Pluronic F 68 at low concentrations. Since the latter surfactant is biologically better accepted, it was favoured in further investigations. The best pilocarpine uptake was obtained with nanoparticles that were purified by washing and ultracentrifugation and dried by lyophilization prior to the adsorption. The optimal Pluronic F 68 concentration for pilocarpine sorption after redispersion of these purified particles was 0.0053 %. A drug loading of about 40 % was thus obtained (Harmia et al., 1986 b).

The adsorption method yielded amorphic particles and no cristallinity was observed by x-ray diffraction. After polymerization in presence of pilocarpine, some cristallinity could be seen. The interesting observation, however, is that some distinct pilocarpine peaks disappear or decrease in intensity in comparison to other peaks as a result of the incorporation. This result may be interpreted in that the cristall structure of pilocarpine after incorporation is different to that of the pure substance (Harmia et al., 1986 a).

The products were then tested in rabbits and the miosis of the rabbit eyes induced by the pilocarpine was registered with a special video system (Harmia et al., 1986 c). The miosis induced by pilocarpine in the form of 2 % normal eye-drop solution lasted for 210 min. The adsorbate prolonged this time to 270 min. The area under the effect-versus-time-curve also was increased by over 30 %. No improvement was obtained with the incorporated products. The improvement in efficacy observed with the adsorbates is comparable to other latex systems.

In conclusion, due to their prolonged persistance in the precorneal area, nanoparticles seem to hold promise for an improvement of the ocular bioavailability of certain drugs. These drugs, however, have to fullfil certain requirements with respect to their physicochemical and probably also to their pharmacodynamic properties.

REFERENCES

Harmia T, Speiser P, Kreuter J (1986 a) A solid colloidal drug delivery system for the eye: encapsulation of pilocarpine in nanoparticles. J Microencapsul 3 : 3-12.

Harmia T, Speiser P, Kreuter J (1986 b) Optimization of pilocarpine loading on to nanoparticles by sorption procedures. Int J Pharm, in press.

Harmia T, Kreuter J, Speiser P, Boye T, Gurny R, Kubis A (1986 c) Enhancement of the myotic response of rabbits with pilocarpine-loaded polybutylcyanoacrylate nanoparticles. Int J Pharm, in press.

Lee VHL, Robinson JR (1979) Mechanistic and quantitative evaluation of precorneal pilocarpine disposition in albino rabbits. J Pharm Sci 68 : 673-684.

Li VHK, Wood RW, Kreuter J, Harmia T, Robinson JR (1986) Ocular drug delivery of progesterone using nanoparticles. J Microencapsul, in press.

Macoul KL, Pavan-Langston D (1975) Pilocarpine ocusert system for sustained control of ocular hypertension. Arch Ophthalmol 93 : 587-590.

Patton TF, Robinson JR (1976) Quantitative precorneal disposition of topically applied pilocarpine nitrate in rabbit eyes. J Pharm Sci 65 : 1295-1301.

Sieg JW, Robinson JR (1979) Vehicle effects on ocular drug bioavailability III. Shear-facilitated pilocarpine release from ointments. J Pharm Sci 68 : 724-728.

Wood RW, Li VHK, Kreuter J, Robinson JR (1985) Ocular disposition of poly-hexyl-2-cyano[3-^{14}C]acrylate nanoparticles in the albino rabbit. Int J Pharm 23 : 175-183.

METHODS TO PRODUCE OCULAR HYPERTENSION IN ANIMALS

L. Bonomi

Istituto di Clinica Oculistica, Università di Verona, Italy

The study of the IOP-lowering effect of drugs in normotensive animal eyes is not a very sensitive method.
For preclinical study of antiglaucoma preparations we developed two simple and reproducible models of experimental ocular hypertension in the rabbit.

A- Transient ocular hypertension is obtained by rapid infusion of 15-20 ml/Kg b.w. of 5% glucose solution into the marginal ear vein.
The eye pressure rapidly increases reaching 26-30 mmHg and then gradually declines. The method has some advantages over water loading by oral gavage and is useful for screening and comparing drugs with possible effect on IOP.

B- A more stable and longer lasting ocular hypertension is induced by repeated weekly subconjunctival injections of 4 mg of a repository preparation of betamethasone. After tne third injection a significant increase of IOP sets in wich is stable for at least 2 weeks.
This allows testing not only the effectiveness of the drugs but also the time course of their effect.

Both models are well reproducible, relatively unexpensive and very sensitive to all kinds of antiglaucoma preparations.

In the search for new medications for glaucoma therapy, potentially interesting drugs must be tested on experimental animals before any clinical trials in human beings are attempted. Unfortunately the effects of drugs on normal IOP is usually slight so that their pressure-lowering properties may be missed or grossly underextimated. The unavoidable tonometric error and physiological and fortuitous IOP fluctuations may act as background noise and interfere with the signal.

This inconvenience becomes particularly important when the matter is the screening of new drugs or the comparison of different drugs or formulations of the same drug.

In the hope of obtaining more reliable results, many models of experimental ocular hypertension have been developed.

Most of them involve extensive trauma to the eye, obvious anatomical changes and other inconveniences. Even the best of them (Gelatt, 1977, Sears and Sears, 1974) have some drawbacks and bear little resemblance to human primary glaucomas.

A very good model in the monkey (Gaasterland and Kupfer, 1974) has given important results in the field of physiopathology, but is too expensive and

Ophthalmic Drug Delivery. Biopharmaceutical, Technological and Clinical Aspects.
M.S. Saettone, G. Bucci, P. Speiser (eds.) Fidia Research Series, vol. 11, Liviana Press, Padova © 1987

scarcely suitable for pharmacological investigations.

In our opinion the requirements for a satisfactory model of ocular hypertension for pharmacological studies are the following.

To leave intact the ocular structures that respond to the action of the drugs; to allow the use of unanesthetized animals therefore normally responsive to drugs and stimuli: to avoid trauma or excessive stimulation of the eye; to be simple, easily reproducible and reasonably unexpensive.

In our laboratory we have developed two models of experimentally raised IOP that meet such requirements.

The animal species choosen is the rabbit: in fact this animal is readily available in large number, is relatively unexpensive, easily handled and lends itself to reproducible tonometries.

The first method is based on the principle of waterloading. Waterdrinking test has been used for many years for the diagnosis of glaucoma.

Waterloading by orogastric gavage has been used as method for increasing IOP in the rabbit (Thorpe and Kolker 1967; Mc Donald et. al., 1969; Seindenhamel and Dungan, 1974). However this method is rather troublesome.

Bietti (1972) has demonstrated that in humans the conventional water load can be advantageously replaced by the intravenous infusion of suitable amounts of 5% glucose solution. This method has the advantage of being simpler and more reproducible than the water-drinking test. Since for reliable tonometry in awake rabbits it is advisable to keep the animals as quiet and unfrightened as possible we thought of adapting this method to the rabbit (Bonomi et. al 1986).

We used New Zealand albino rabbits, of about 3 Kg of body weight, coming from the same breed.

Different amounts of glucose solution were injected through a 20-gauge needle into the marginal vein of the ear, taking care that in all animals the infusion was accomplished within 20 seconds.

Tonometries were performed by means of a Mckay-Marg electronic tonometer under surface anesthesia (0.4% benoxinate).

Immediately after the end of infusion the eye pressure increased in all animals, reaching its maximun level between 5 and 10 minutes and returning to pretreatment levels within 40 minutes. The values of IOP increase were dependent on the aumont of solution infused: the administration of 15 ml/Kg b.w. produced an increase of about 10 mmHg, whereas with 10 and 5 ml/Kg b.w. a still clear but quantitatively less important effect was reached (Fig. 1).

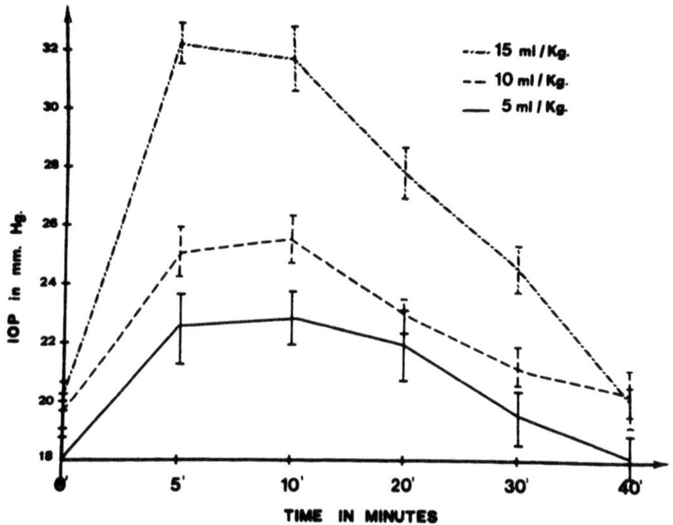

Figure 1
Mean IOP in 18 rabbits after the intravenous infusion of different amounts of 5% glucose solution.

The values and the course of the ocular pressure elevation were superposable in the two eyes so that it is possible to treat with a given drug one eye using the contralateral for comparison. In some instances the drug may influence also the contralateral eye; in this case the comparison is made with a second group of control animals.

The model is sensitive to all kinds of drugs active on the IOP and it has been used in our laboratory for testing many antiglaucoma medications. The differences in pressure between treated and control eyes are much more evident during the course of the ocular hypertension than in normotensive eyes. (Fig. 2 and 3)

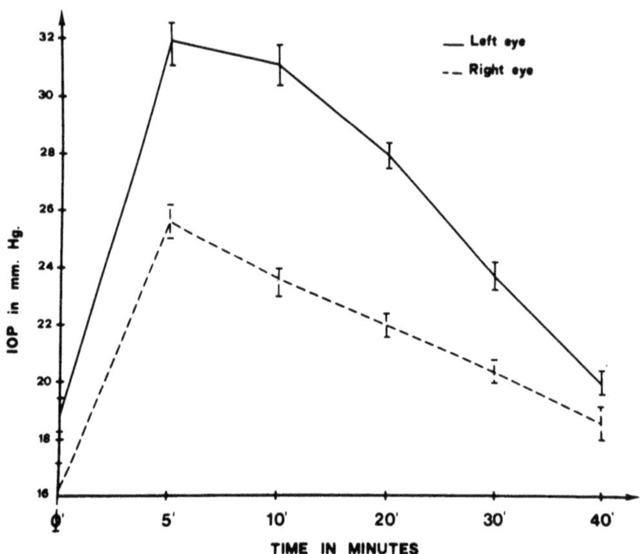

Figure 2
IOP course in 6 rabbits after infusion of 15 ml/Kg b.w. of 5% glucose solution. The right eyes were treated with 2% pilocarpine.

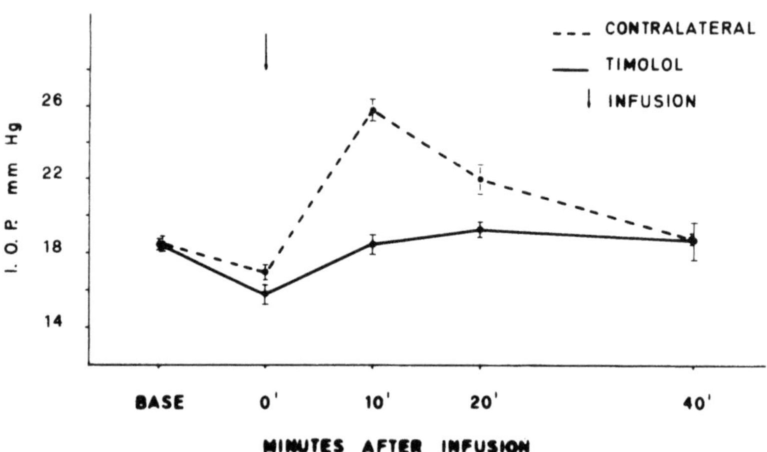

Figure 3.
Effect of the instillation of 0.5% timolol in 6 rabbits (infusion model).

The method is simple, well reproducible and easy to perform. We made statistics on 504 rabbits used in a series of experiments: only the 0.4% of the animals died during the test and only 5% failed to show a satisfactory ocular hypertension. The mean IOP at the 10th minute from the end of the infusion was 26±1.91 mmHg.

The method is suitable for screening work and for comparing the effect of drugs but, due to the short duration of the ocular hypertension, cannot be used for the evaluation of the duration of the drug effect.

We have also developed a second model that allows more complete results. Corticosteroid glaucoma in humans is probably the form of secondary glaucoma that most closely resembles the spontaneous illness of the open-angle type.

So far attempts at increasing IOP in rabbits by topical or systemic corticosteroid administration have either failed or produced transient and ill-reproducible results with important systemic side effects and high rates of morbidity and mortality (Liebe, 1963; Tuovinen et al., 1966; Tarkkanen et al., 1967; Levene et al.; Lorenzetti,1970; Virno et al., 1974; Wood et al. 1967).

Nevertheless it is clear that the rabbit eye responds to corticosteroid treatment if high local administrations of the drug are maintained for sufficient time. The incosistency of the results may be interpreted as due to the serious decay in the general conditions of the animals as a consequence of the large systemic absorption of the drug. Since local injections of repository forms of corticosteroids allow high local concentrations for a long time with little spreading of the drug into general circulation, we believed that the obstacle could be overcome by using this way of administration.

New Zealand albino rabbits weighing about 3 Kg were subjected to subconjunctival injections of 0.8 ml of Bentelan Depot (Glaxo) corresponding to 4 mg of betamethasone. The injections were repeated weekly for three weeks.

After the first week a slight but real increase of IOP was observed. After the third injection IOP was over 26 mmHg and it remained stable for further 2 weeks (fig. 4).

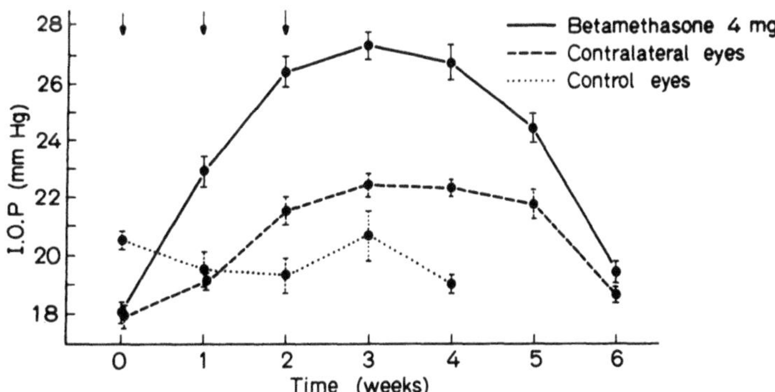

Figure 4.

Time course of IOP in rabbits subjected to 3 subconjunctival injections of repository betamethasone.

A slighter increase of IOP was present also in the contralateral eye. Lower dosages of the corticosteroid induced insufficient effects. Larger dosages produced important systemic effects with evident decay of the animals and death of many of them.

The systemic administration of the same dosage of the steroid failed to induce any ocular hypertension.

We observed that IOP courses in consecutive days of the third week were perfectly superposable (fig. 5).

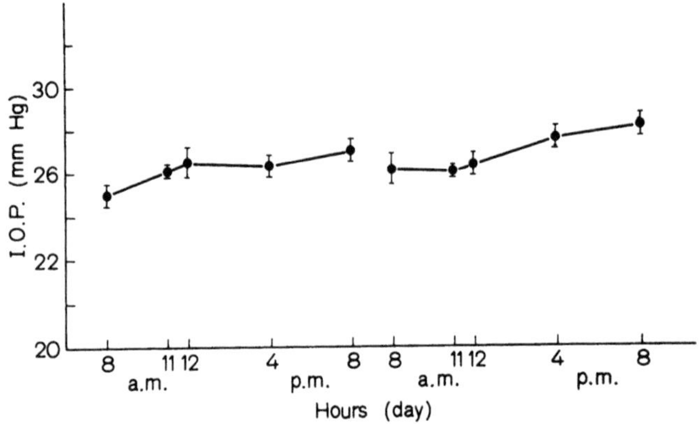

Figure 5.
IOP curve during two consecutive days (23 and 24) in 6 rabbits with betamethasone ocular hypertension.

This make possible to evaluate the effects of drugs using as baseline the measurements of the preceding day. This allows also the evaluation of the duration of the tensional effect of a single dose. On the contrary a comparison with the contralateral eyes of the same animals is not possible (Bonomi et al., 1978).

Also this method is very sensitive to the action of the different kinds of antiglaucoma medications.

We used it with good results for the study of several drugs (fig. 6 and 7).

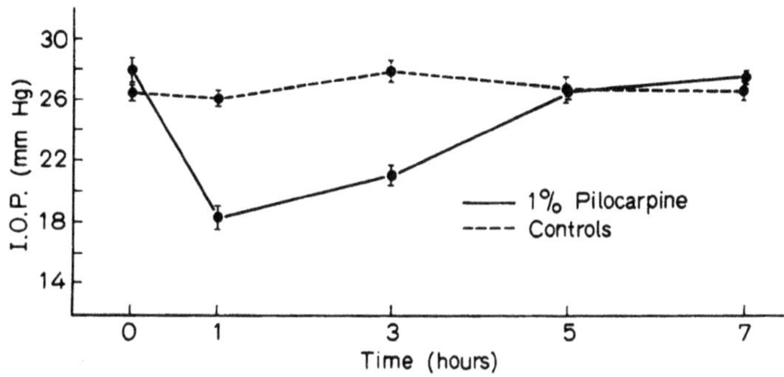

Figure 6.
Effect of a single instillation of 1% pilocarpine in 6 rabbits with betamethasone ocular hypertension.

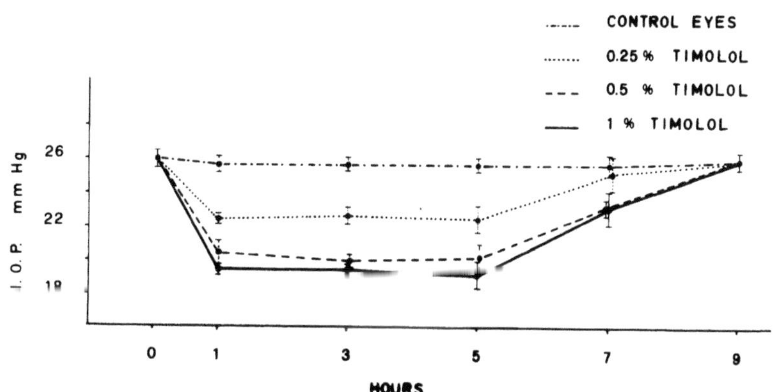

Figure 7.
Effects of 3 different concentrations of timolol on the betamethasone ocular hypertension of the rabbit.

This method is very useful and fairly well reproducible. We made statistics on 764 rabbits used in a large series of experiments and found the following data: only 12% of the animals failed to develop a satisfactory ocular hypertension while only 8% of the animals died during the experiment.

In the remaining rabbits the mean IOP at the third week was 27.46±2.12 mmHg.

After the publication in 1978 of our corticosteroid model we were informed that several investigators had not been succesful in reproducing it in their laboratories. We tried to identifie the reasons of these failures and reached the following conclusions. The body weight of the animals is important; it should be not less than 3 Kg. the conditions of stabulation are of utmost importance: the temperature must be kept constantly around 16° Centrigrades, the humidifaction must be good and the lighting not excessive. Unnecessary noise must also be avoided.

The use of McKag-Marg tonometer is advisable.

The tonometric technique must be correct and avoid damage to the corneal epithelium which can lead to erroneous readings.

The two methods allow a reasonably reliable preclinical experimentation of antiglaucoma drugs. A direct transposition of the results to the human field is obviously impossible. However the results obtained with our models are generally in good agreement with the effects of the drugs in the human eye as shown in Table 1. The different distribution of the adrenergic receptors in the rabbit and primate eyes may explain the discrepancies found in the evaluation of drugs active on the alpha-receptors.

TABLE 1.

PERCENT DECREASE OF INTRAOCULAR PRESSURE

		5% Glucose	Betamethasone Ocular Hypertension	Human open angle glaucoma
1%	Pilocarpine	24-28	30	20-30
1%	Epinephrine	25	20	15-30
0.5%	Timolol	28	24	20-38
1%	Propranolol	22	20	17
1%	Pindolol	25	25	25
0.5%	Labetalol	28	22	21
1%	Thymoxamine	18	30	14
0.125%	Clonidine	20	25	16

REFERENCES

Bietti GB (1972) Recent experimental clinical and therapeutic research on the problems of intraocular pressure and glaucoma. Am.J. Ophthal. 73: 475.

Bonomi L, Perfetti S, Noja E, Bellucci R, Tomazzoli L (1978) Experimental corticosteroid ocular hypertension in the rabbit. Graefes Arch. Klin. Exp. Ophthal. 209: 73

Bonomi L, Tomazzoli L, Jaria D (1976) An improved model of experimentally induced ocular hypertension in the rabbit. Invest Ophthalmol. 15: 781

Gaasterland D, Kupfer C (1974) Experimental glaucoma in the Rhesus monkey. Invest. Ophthalmol. 13: 455

Gelatt KN (1977) Animal models for glaucoma. Invest. Ophthalmol. 16: 592

Levene RZ, Rothberg M, Rosemberg S (1974) Corticosteroids glaucoma in the rabbit. Am. J. Ophthal. 78: 505

Lieb W (1963) Changes in the dynamics of the aqueous humor on account of influences exerted on the mucopolysaccharide metabolism. Klin. Monatsbl. Augenhelkd 142:982

Lorenzetti OJ (1970) Effect of corticosteroids on ocular dynamics in rabbits. J. Phar. Exp. Ther. 175: 763

McDonald TO, Hodges JW, Borgmann AR (1969) The water-loading test in rabbits. Arch. Ophthal. 82: 381

Sears D, Sears M (1974) Blood-aqueous barrier and alpha-chymotrypsin glaucoma in rabbits. Am.J. Ophthal. 77: 070

Seidenhamel RG, Dungan KW (1974) Characteristc and pharmacologic utility of an intraocular pressure (IOP) model in unanesthetized rabbits. Invest. Ophthal. 13: 319

Tarkkanen A, Esila R, Tenhunen T (1967) Ocular effects of long-term parenteral administration of triamcinolone. Ann. Chir. Gynaecol. 56: 467

Thorpe RM, Kolker AE (1967) A tonographic study of water loading in rabbits. Arch. Ophthal. 77: 238

Tuovinen E, Esila R, Liesmaa M (1966) The influence of corticosteroids on intraocular pressure in rabbits. I. The influence of massive intramuscular doses of cortisone and prednisolone. Acta Ophthal. 44: 581

Tuovinen E, Esila R, Liesmaa (1966) The influence corticosteroids on intraocular pressure in rabbits. II. The influence of massive subconjunctival doses of dexamethasone and betamethasone. Acta Ophthal. 44: 901

Tuovinen E, Esila R, Liesmaa M (1966) The influence or corticosteroids on intraocular pressure in rabbits. III. The immediate influence of massive intravenous doses of betamethasone and dexamethasone on the intraocular pressure of the rabbit eye. Acta Ophthal. 44: 823

Virno M, Schirru A, Pecori-Girardi J, Pellegrino N (1974) Aqueous humor alkalosis and marked reduction in ocular ascorbic acid content following long-term topical cortisone (9 a-fluoro-16-a-methylprednisolone). Ann. Ophthal. 6: 983

Wood DC, Contaxis I, Sweet D, Smith JC, Van Dolah J (1967) Responsens of rabbit to corticosteroids. I. Influence on growth, intraocular pressure and lens trasparency. Am.J. Ophthal. 63: 841

PHARMACOKINETICS AND BIOPHARMACEUTICAL ASPECTS OF SOME ANTI-GLAUCOMA DRUGS

B. Plazonnet, J. Grove, M. Durr, C. Mazuel, M. Quint and A. Rozier

Merck Sharp & Dohme-Chibret, Centre de Recherche
Route de Marsat, 63203 Riom, France

The therapy of glaucoma has used several classes of active ingredients which were mostly cholinergic and adrenergic drugs. The carbonic anhydrase inhibitors were essentially systemic drugs but recently new potent compounds have been described to be active after topical administration. Each class of drugs has a different pharmacokinetic behaviour due to the physico-chemical properties of the individual compounds. The dynamics of ocular fluids, especially the turnover of tears, are responsible for a poor availability of drugs administered topically in the conjunctival cul-de-sac. The recent galenic developments in ophthalmic formulations have essentially aimed at achieving better control of the residence of anti-glaucoma drugs close to the anterior segment of the eye and derivatization and prodrug approaches have improved transcorneal penetration.

INTRODUCTION

Anti-glaucoma drugs are the most widely prescribed class of ophthalmics. They are almost always administered locally. Like other topical ophthalmics, they are subject to the constraints of the dynamics of ocular fluids and eye tissue barriers. Various classes of drugs are used for glaucoma, but essentially they all reduce intra-ocular pressure by decreasing aqueous humor formation and/or increasing aqueous humor elimination. Recently, carbonic anhydrase inhibitors (CAIs) which were previously administered exclusively by the systemic route have been re-examined and new compounds as well as new formulations have been proposed for their topical application. It will be interesting to see if the acquired knowledge of ocular pharmacokinetics and of recent ophthalmic formulations can be transferred successfully to the design of formulations for topically active CAIs.

This review will deal successively with general considerations, animal models, viscosity, pilocarpine, adrenergic drugs and carbonic anhydrase inhibitors.

1. GENERAL CONSIDERATIONS OF OCULAR TOPICAL THERAPY.

The fate of any medicine can be divided sequentially into three phases : a pharmaceutical phase, a pharmacokinetic phase and a pharmacodynamic phase

Ophthalmic Drug Delivery. Biopharmaceutical, Technological and Clinical Aspects.
M.S. Saettone, G. Bucci, P. Speiser (eds.) Fidia Research Series, vol. 11, Liviana Press, Padova © 1987

(Ariens, 1974). Topical ophthalmics are unique in this scheme because the pharmaceutical formulation administered is very close to the receptor site. The pharmacokinetic phase which usually encompasses absorption, distribution, metabolism and excretion is less important; whereas the pharmaceutical phase, which determines the availability of drug for absorption, plays a critical role. The constituents of the formulation will modify the quality of the contact with the anterior segment of the eye and the residence and the rate of penetration in the ocular tissues. Moreover, the ophthalmic vehicle administered to this very sensitive organ should be completely innocuous.

A number of reviews have been published recently which reinforce these considerations or draw the attention to specific points. Besides the publication edited by Robinson (1980), there are papers by Mishima (1981), Maurice & Mishima (1984), Sears (1984), Shell (1982), Shell (1984), McLaughlin & Chiou (1985), Burnstein & Anderson (1985), Buri (1985), Lee & Robinson (1986). These reviews contain numerous references. In addition, an earlier paper by Benson (1974) should be consulted.

A very simplified approximation to describe the access of antiglaucoma drugs to their site(s) of action is through trans-corneal passive diffusion, governed by the lipophilic-hydrophilic characteristics of the compounds, (Lee et al, 1982). Since at physiological pH, available anti-glaucoma agents are essentially weak bases, they are largely ionized i.e. more soluble in aqueous media. The main barrier is thus the corneal epithelium which favors the penetration of lipid soluble entities (Camber, 1985, Mindel et al, 1984). Non-corneal routes of ocular penetration, although of little significance for those drugs known at present (Doane et al, 1978), have been recently reinvestigated by Ahmed & Patton (1985) for timolol and inulin.

These authors have shown that, when corneal access was blocked in the albino rabbit, a 25 µl instillation of 0.65% ^{14}C-timolol induced at 20 minutes, iris + ciliary body levels that were 13% of those obtained when corneal access was free. In contrast, using ^{14}C-inulin under the same conditions, the iris + ciliary body levels without corneal access were 80% of those obtained with corneal penetration. Hence, non-corneal penetration routes might be more important when the lipophilic-hydrophilic balance does not favor transcorneal penetration.

Although the local route is usually far superior to systemic dosage, the topical drug applied onto the eye in a drop yields low ocular concentrations. This poor ocular bioavailability after local administration is due to the corneal barrier and ocular fluid dynamics. The most significant area where drug losses occur is the precorneal area. The amount of drug entering the precorneal tear film area after instillation is drastically decreased before it can reach its locus of action e.g. the triggering site(s) for secretion and/or excretion of the aqueous humor (Lee & Robinson, 1986). Following instillation, the vehicle is drained by reflex blinking and tear secretion, (Chrai et al, 1974, Zaki et al, 1986, Ludwig & Van Ooteghem, 1986a). In addition to a variable decrease from tear formation (vide infra), the concentration of the active ingredient is also decreased by absorption into the surrounding ocular tissues (e.g. conjunctivae), by tear protein binding, (Mikkelson et al, 1973) and metabolism.

2. ABOUT RABBITS AND MEN

Most of our knowledge of the fate of ophthalmic drugs as well as the influence of parameters on the formulation has been obtained through animal experiments, primarily in the albino rabbit. Indeed, the rabbit has been used in experimental ophthalmology since the 17th century (Prince 1964). An understanding of the physiology of the eye, the similarities and the differences between the the rabbit and man is therefore of the utmost importance. The pharmaceutical implications of these differences have been reviewed recently by Lee & Robinson (1986). They conclude that there are three main points of difference :- the precorneal area, the presence of a nictitating membrane and the lack of melanin pigments. Schlem's canal is not apparent in rabbits and in man uveoscleral drainage might be more important. Otherwise, under normal conditions, differences in volume, turnover rate and chemical constitution of the aqueous humors of the two species seem to be of minimal importance.

In the precorneal area, although the tear volume ca 7 µl is identical, the tear turnover rate is approximately 7% per minute in rabbit and 16% in man. The composition of the tear film can vary, for example, the rabbit tear film can be richer in lipids (Holly & Lemp, 1973). The maximum quantity of fluid that can be contained in the human cul-de-sac without overflow is about 30 µl (Mishima, 1966, 1981). The albino rabbit can accomodate, with careful instillation, volumes up to 50 µl (the conjunctival pouches of the beagle dog and of the rhesus monkey are by far smaller). Drop size is discussed later in the paper. A major difference between rabbits and man is the frequency of blinking, which can be 2-4 per hour in rabbits and approximately 12 per minute in man. The net result of differences in tear turnover rates and blinking frequency is a solution drainage rate constant estimated to be $0.545/min^{-1}$ in rabbit and $1.45/min^{-1}$ in man (Lee & Robinson, 1986). Recent studies on the influence of the vehicle on ^{99m}Tc disposition in the precorneal area have confirmed that in man the instilled material is more rapidly removed than in rabbit.

The existence of a nictitating membrane in rabbits leads to stagnation of very viscous solutions between it and the cornea in the lower inner quadrant of the anterior segment. Accumulation of some drugs can occur in the membrane i.e. epinephrine (Anderson, 1980). On the other hand, the removal of this third lid did not modify the absorption kinetics of pilocarpine and epinephrine after topical instillation. (De Santis & Schoenwald, 1978 and Mindel et al (1984).

The iris and ciliary body of the albino rabbit does not contain melanin. Lyons & Krohn (1964) and Lee & Robinson (1982), among others, have reported the high binding capacity of the uveal tissues of the pigmented rabbit for anti-glaucoma drugs. The pigmented rabbit eye can also exhibit a higher enzymatic activity than the albino eye especially for pilocarpine (Lee 1983, Lee et al 1985), although pilocarpic acid has also been found in the aqueous humor of albino rabbits (Plazonnet & Cerdeno, 1976). The response to the ß-blocker timolol can vary with pigmentation (Katz & Berger 1979). Enzymatic activities found in ocular tissues are, catechol-O-methyltransferase, monoamine oxidase, steroid 6-ßhydroxylase, oxidoreductase, lysosomal enzymes, esterases, peptidases, glucuronide and sulfate transferase and glutathione conjugating enzymes (Lee et al, 1985).

A steroidal 17-21 desmolase activity has also been reported (Ono et al, 1971, Hamard et al, 1975). If inter-animal variability of this desmolase occurs, this might explain the poor reproducibility of the induction of ocular hypertension in rabbits by potent corticosteroids.

3. VISCOSITY OF FORMULATIONS

After a hypothetical instantaneous perfect mixing (between an instillate and tear fluids), any active ingredient in solution is removed from the precorneal area by the tear drainage. In man, the theoretical time for complete removal of the compound is approximately 7 minutes, during which time the tear fluid concentration is decreased exponentially (Robinson, 1980). Increasing the viscosity of the ophthalmic vehicle has been a long-accepted procedure aimed at reducing the drainage rate. Since there is practically no ointment formulation of anti-glaucoma drugs in the current practice, only aqueous solutions whose viscosity has been increased with a water-soluble/dispersible polymer will be considered. The viscosity of such formulations can be varied from a few centipoises to a gel. The common consensus is that polymers in solutions, e.g. polyvinyl alcohol, cellulose derivatvives, polyvinylpyrolidone or dextran derivatives, increase viscosity and induce a better spreading on the anterior segment and improved mixing with the tear film. This reduces drainage and prolongs to some extent the initial tear concentration of the drug, yielding better bioavailability, possible sustained release and less frequent dosing (Adler et al, 1971, Benedetto et al, 1975). The investigation of the role of viscosity and the equivalence or inequivalence of various polymers has been a field where animal experiments have been used extensively (Chrai & Robinson, 1974). However, the clinical relevance of the findings is regularly questioned. It has been claimed that an increase of viscosity of an instillate greater than 15 - 20 centipoises would not increase ocular bioavailability in man. (Patton & Robinson, 1975, Eriksen, 1980).

Recently, non-invasive methods have allowed the influence of various vehicles on precorneal disposition to be studied without sampling of tears. Ludwig & Van Ooteghem (1986a) have re-examined the in situ fluorophotometric decay of sodium fluorescein previously reported by Adler at al (1971) and Benedetto et al (1975). Gamma scintigraphy has been employed by the group at Nottingham, UK, (Wilson et al, 1983, Olijnik et al, 1983 and Zaki et al, 1986), to reinvestigate the role of viscosity, the nature of the polymer, and compare the behaviour of the viscous formulations in rabbit and man. Their data confirm those of Saettone and co-workers who, using biological indexes (miosis or mydriasis), found that not only the viscosity, but also the polymer itself, modified bio-availability of ophthalmic drugs (Saettone et al, 1982, 1984).

These two groups also concur in finding that the rabbit is less sensitive than man to moderate increases of formulation viscosity (Saettone et al, 1982, Saettone et al, 1986, Zaki et al, 1986). This conclusion is essentially the same as that of Benedetto et al (1985) and Melis-Decerf and Van Ooteghem (1979), although Van Ooteghem (1983) reported that prolonged action might be more easily shown in rabbit when viscosity was increased.

Aqueous gels are at the upper limit of viscous preparations. Gels are formed when high molecular weight polymers and/or high polymer concentrations are incorporated into the formulation. Under this definition, the product pre-exists as a gel before administration. Preparations which are practically non-viscous liquids in the dispenser and turn into gels in the conjunctival cul-de-sac due to changes in environmental conditions, i.e. temperature, pH etc.. are known. Investigations on gel formation by change of temperature have been described (Vadnere et al, 1984). Ophthalmic gels of commercial and experimental use will be mentioned later in this paper.

Bioadhesion has recently been advanced as an approach to longer residence times of ophthalmic formulations without the traditional use of viscosifying agents. The basic postulate is that due to conformation and anionic charges, some polymers specifically bind to mucins e.g. from the conjunctiva (Park & Robinson, 1981, Hui & Robinson, 1985, Robert & Buri, 1986, Lee & Robinson 1986 and references therein). This concept of bioadhesion has been put forward to explain the role and the potential interest of poly (alkyl-cyanoacrylates), nanoparticles and Piloplex (vide infra).

4. DROP SIZE

The effect of the drop size on ocular drainage has been the subject of a series of investigations (Chrai et al, 1973, 1974). Patton and Robinson (1976) concluded that when the same amount of drug was used, a smaller drop of a higher concentration delivered the compound more effectively than a larger drop of smaller concentration. This was confirmed in laboratory and published work (Patton, 1977, Patton 1980, Ludwig & Van Ooteghem 1986b). In man, the size of an administered drop is limited by the capacity of the conjunctival fornix (Sugaya & Nagataki, 1978, Mishima et al, 1966, File & Patton, 1980) and by the reflex blinking after instillation (Maurice & Mishima, 1984). The importance of drop size of various commercial products has been specifically addressed recently for some anti-glaucoma drugs by Lederer & Harold (1986), Brown et al (1985). The size of the delivered drop of an ophthalmic drug is frequently grossly exaggerated and is no longer 70 µl as often suggested. For example, Timoptic® and Timoptol® Ocumeters™ deliver constant volume drops of 31 ± 1 µl drops, essentially because of 0.01% benzalkonium choride, a common anti-microbial preservative which decreases drop size by decreasing surface tension. Frequent attempts have been made to obtain the delivery of a uniform and consistent small drop to the patients' eye.

Part of the rationale for the use of smaller drops is the belief that they might reduce the frequency and/or intensity of the side effects of ophthalmic drugs (Brown & Lynch, 1986). This has not yet been definitively established. The reduction of side effects might also be attained through modifications of ophthalmic drugs and formulations to obtain better local bioavailibility and a sustained effect. For instance, Chang et al (1986a) have recently claimed that a prodrug of timolol would be a better approach than decreasing the drop size to reduce the systemic load after topical ocular timolol administration (vide infra).

5. RECENT ADVANCES IN PILOCARPINE DELIVERY

Pilocarpine is the "oldest" anti-glaucoma drug; numerous different formulations are marketed. It has been observed that every time a new matrix or a new polymer formulation has been discovered or an ingenious drug delivery device invented, it has been subsequently applied to topical ocular administration of pilocarpine in the rabbit.

From a vast and diversified collection of pharmaceutical forms of pilocarpine, the following are of special interest: the soluble ophthalmic inserts (SODI & other matrices) described by Maichuck (1975), Yakovlev & Lenkevich (1966), Katz and Blackman (1977), Saettone & et al (1984b), Urtti (1985), Urtti et al (1985a,b), the Alza Ocusert® (Shell & Baker, 1974, Urquhart 1980, Heilman 1984), the pilocarpine alginate (Loucas & Haddad, 1976). An aqueous gel and the emulsified systems have pioneered several interesting approaches to viable systems, whereas the soft contact lenses soaked in pilocarpine solutions (Waltman & Kaufman, 1970, Podos et al, 1972, Eller et al, 1985) remained only experimental tools. Carbomer gel (Pilopine) is an aqueous gel containing 4% pilocarpine hydrochloride (Schoenwald et al 1978,, Ellis et al, 1985, Aldrete et al, 1983, March et al, 1982). Administration at bedtime allows a 24-hour control of intraocular pressure and of side effects such as miosis (March et al, 1982). Induction of myopia and changes in refraction occur when the patient is sleeping. Polyoxy-ethylene glycol and methyl cellulose gels of Pilocarpine have been compared with an ointment (Habib et al, 1985). In the rabbit, they found that the gels gave a better IOP response than the ointment and they related this to better mixing and dissolution of the aqueous vehicles compared to the oily base.

Considering that aqueous suspensions can give improved bioavailability due to some of the particles escaping from the normal drainage of the lacrimal fluids (Sieg & Robinson, 1965, Sieg & Triplett, 1980), it might be of interest to have pilocarpine formulated as a suspension or an emulsion. Recent developments in this area are Piloplex, nanoparticles and latex. Piloplex is an aqueous emulsion of a pilocarpine salt of a polymeric anion. This anion is based on a basic unit formed from acrylic acid and lauryl methacrylate (U.S. patent 4,248,855, Blumenthal et al, 1976, Ticho et al, 1979a,b, Anderman et al, 1983, Klein et al, 1985). It was published that a formulation equivalent to 3.4% of pilocarpine allowed a b.i.d. regimen (Ticho et al, 1979a,b). Piloplex precipitates and coagulates in the cul-de-sac due to changes in the ionic environment, then pilocarpine is slowly released from this coagulum which persists for a long time by virtue of bioadhesion. The results obtained in rabbits by Robinson & Li (1984) are consistent with the clinical findings cited above. The presence of a lauryl radical aids emulsification of this polymer salt but adequate stability is not attained due to the neutral pH of the emulsion (Kreienbaum & Page, 1986, Dunn et al, 1981, Kennedy & McNamara, 1981, Noordam et al, 1978, Urbanyi et al, 1976).

Another approach toward a dispersed system is the preparation of nanoparticles. These are colloidal particles, 10-1000 nm in size, in which a drug such as a pilocarpine salt may be dispersed, encapsulated, and/or adsorbed. The drug release may then be controlled either by the capsule wall or by the particle matrix (Chieu, 1978). The dispersions described by

Kreuter (1983a,b) have been used for pilocarpine. Butylcyanoacrylate was polymerized in an acidic solution of pilocarpine containing Pluronic F68 as an emulsifier and then brought to neutrality (Harmia et al, 1986a). Entrapment of pilocarpine nitrate can reach 60%, giving a final concentration of ca 0.1 mg per 10 μl, which induced a sustained pharmacological effect in the rabbit (Harmia et al, 1986b). Similar nanoparticles made from hexyl-2-cyanoacrylate were studied in rabbit by Wood et al (1985) using radiotracer techniques. They found that the nanoparticles were rapidly removed by drainage from the precorneal area. However, the retention of the nanoparticles was better than that of drug solution possibly through bioadhesion to cornea and conjunctiva, or to the structural features of the polymer. Nanoparticles are certainly of experimental interest, although their use as a vehicle for ocular drug delivery has two limitations. Firstly, the coefficient of entrapment can be rather low and secondly, the intrinsic stability of the ester i.e. its tendency to hydrolyse in neutral aqueous media, can hamper its pharmaceutical use. For the moment, only freeze-dried preparations requiring reconstitution before their administration would appear practical.

Another sustained release system is the latex formulation developed by Gurny et al (1980, 1981a,b, 1985). In contrast to the previous systems, pilocarpine is dissolved in the continuous phase (aqueous) in which 30% insoluble polymer (cellulose acetate phthallate) is dispersed as submicron particles (ca 0.3 μm). The pH of this latex, about 4.5, creates conditions for the stability of the system. Upon instillation, the tears buffer the formulation to around 7 thereby inducing coagulation of the polymer. This quasi-matrix entraps the drug which is subsequently released slowly as the polymer dissolves. When a latex was compared to an equivalent isotonic solution of 4% pilocarpine HCl in rabbits, the AUC of the miosis curve of the former exhibited a 50% increase, in addition, the peak effect was delayed (Gurny et al, 1985). It can be speculated that a b.i.d. regimen in patients should be possible with this preparation. The latex pH of 4.5 is adequate to prevent hydrolysis of pilocarpine, and a stable formulation would be anticipated. The buffering capacity of tears has to exceed the buffering capacity of the polymer to optimize tolerance and availability of pilocarpine (Mitra & Mikkelson, 1982).

A radically different approach relies on the formation of prodrugs of pilocarpine. Bundgaard et al (1985, 1986a,b,c) have studied an extensive list of mono- and diesters of pilocarpic acid. Various benzyl pilocarpates which are hydrolyzed enzymatically and then lactonized by pH-mediated equilibrium looked promising (Bundgaard et al, 1986c). Unfortunately mono-esterified pilocarpates had too short a half-life to be useful in ophthalmic formulations. Diesters, such as O-phenyl pilocarpic acid benzyl ester or O-butyryl pilocarpic acid 4-methylbenzyl ester, at pHs of 4 - 5, had a calculated shelf life far larger than the parent drug. Experimental measurements of miosis in rabbits appear very encouraging for these diesters (Bundgaard, 1986). The main drawback of the prodrugs is that from a developmental stand point, they are new chemical and drug entities. Hence, the process of producing a marketable product can be tedious and lengthy.

6. ADRENERGIC DRUGS

The major advance in glaucoma therapy during the late seventies was the introduction of timolol maleate (Timoptic®, Timoptol®), a potent non-selective ß-blocker, to treat chronic open-angle glaucoma (Zimmerman & Kaufman 1977, Vareilles et al, 1977, 1978). As a result, considerable interest has been devoted to the potential of any ß-adrenergic drug for the topical treatment of glaucoma (Sears, 1981, Lotti et al, 1984a, McLaughlin & Chiou 1985). The numerous ß-blockers used and/or tested in cardio-vascular pharmacology has permitted comparisons between their structure, activity and pharmacokinetics when topically applied in the eye. In a series of papers, Schoenwald & Huang (1983), Huang et al (1983a,b) have examined the corneal penetration of ß-blocking agents by in-vitro measurements with excised rabbit corneas. They studied twelve ß-adrenergic agents having octanol/water partition coefficients over a 4-fold logarithmic range. For eleven of these compounds, they established a correlation between the corneal permeability coefficient and the distribution coefficient (DC). They also estimated the respective contribution of epithelium, stroma and endothelium from experimentally determined permeability coefficients (Huang et al, 1983a) The table below has been constructed to summarize their data.

Table 1

		% CONTRIBUTION OF INDIVIDUAL CORNEAL LAYERS		
	LOG (DC) RANGE	EPITHELIUM	STROMA	ENDOTHELIUM
HYDROPHILIC	(-0.52 - 0.2)	94.6 ± 2.7	0.9 ± 0.3	4.5 ± 2.5
LIPOPHILIC	(0.28 - 0.72)	54.8 ± 10.4	15.8 ± 9.5	29.5 ± 5.5
VERY LIPOPHILIC	(1.68 - 2.53)	8.3 ± 7.1	46.3 ± 2.6	45.5 ± 9.3
OVERALL		**52.5 ± 37.5**	**20.9 ± 20.0**	**26.50 ± 18.5**

Mean ± S.D.; N = 4, calculated from data of Huang et al 1983a.

From the above, it can be seen that epithelium resistance decreased by an order of magnitude for the very lipophilic compounds. Overall, the importance of epithelium resistance is emphasized by the fact that it is practically equal to the sum of the stromal and endothelial contributions. Studies correlating in-vitro and in-vivo data obtained in rabbit with three drugs ranging from lipophilic (bufuralol) to hydrophilic (acebutolol) through timolol, led them to conclude that peak time was inversely related to corneal permeability and that the "most lipophilic" agents bufuralol and timolol did not behave as predicted for C max and AUC. Aqueous boundary layers were postulated to describe *in-vivo* corneal permeability which, in turn, would imply that bufuralol and timolol may have essentially the same ocular permeability coefficients in rabbits (Huang *et al*, 1983b). There are five important topical ß-blockers currently used in ophthalmology, namely Timolol, Metipranolol, Carteolol, Betaxolol and Levobunolol. Due to their high potency, they are prescribed in low concentrations (0.1 - 2%), and are formulated in simple buffered solutions. The dosing regimen is usually b.i.d., which is convenient, both physicians and patients being apparently well satisfied with these formulations.

Until recently, modifications of ß-blocking drugs and/or their formulations to increase efficacity have rarely been attempted. Harmia-Pulkinnen *et al* (1986) have described the manufacture of alkylcyano-acrylate nanoparticles with timolol. Bundgaard *et al* (1986) prepared acetyl, propionyl, butyryl and pivaloyl esters of timolol and measured the relative increase of corneal penetration compared to underivatized timolol. The enhanced lipophilicity of these esters induced a higher corneal permeablity *in-vitro* and timolol was regenerated by the ocular tissues. The prodrug, the O-butyryl ester of timolol exhibited a corneal permeability that was increased by a factor of 3.3 when compared to an equivalent dose of timolol (Kaila *et al*, 1985, Bundgaard *et al*, 1986, Chang *et al*, 1986b). The same group (Chang *et al*, 1986a,b) demonstrated that 80% of a 25 µl dose of 1% timolol was absorbed systemically and that the use of chondroitin sulfate used as a vehicle enhanced both ocular and systemic absorption. They also showed that O-butyryl timolol increased ocular absorption by a factor of 6 to 8 without significantly affecting the systemic absorption. Unfortunately, these esters were rapidly hydrolyzed in solution thus leading to very short shelf lives. Formulations and/or structural changes in the molecules which will reduce plasma concentrations of ophthalmic ß-blockers will probably emerge in the near future.

Dipivaloyl epinephrine (McClure, 1975) is another example of the successful design of a prodrug (Krause, 1980). The object was to increase ocular bioavailability through changes in lipophicity, thereby increasing the corneal permeation.

DIPIVEFRIN EPINEPHRINE

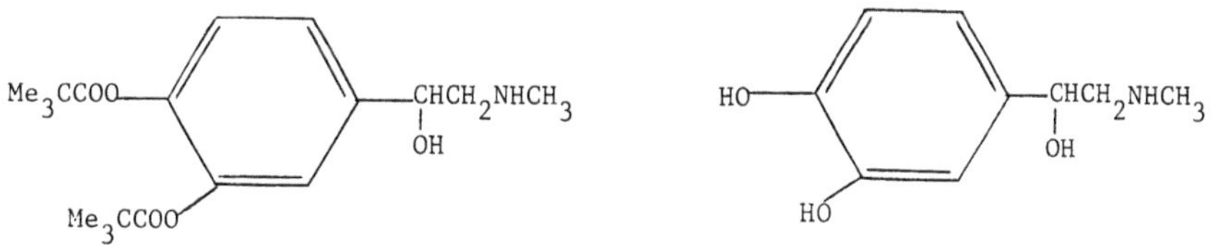

Me_3CCOO — $CHCH_2NHCH_3$ (OH) ; Me_3CCOO

HO — $CHCH_2NHCH_3$ (OH) ; HO

0.0081 DC 4.89

n-octanol/buffered saline pH 7.2

The ratio of the partition coefficients of the ester and epinephrine (~600) explains why 17 times more dipivaloyl epinephrine penetrates the cornea than epinephrine (Wei *et al*, 1978, Mandell *et al*, 1978). Grass & Robinson (1984) claimed the viscosity of a formulation would have little effect on a drug with a partition coefficient greater than 10. They suggested that drugs with higher lipophilicity partition easily into the corneal epithelium and any transient increase in pre-corneal residence time due to the viscosity of the vehicle would be of negligible effect. Although not greater than 10, the partition coefficient of dipivefrin is the same order of magnitude and changes considerably the status of dipivaloyl epinephrine vis à vis corneal penetration. The most active site of hydrolysis of a prodrug is the rabbit cornea, (Krause, 1980), which is of interest as a general guideline during the development of new compounds via the prodrug approach (vide infra). Mandell et al (1978) and Anderson et al (1980) have published data on intraocular levels of epinephrine after administration of the two compounds, epinephrine and dipivaloyl epinhephrine in albino rabbits. Anderson et al (1980) give the following data :-

Table 2

	RATIO (DIPIVEFRIN / EPINEPHRINE)*		
TIME / TISSUE	30 MIN	60 MIN	3 HR
CORNEA	19.6	14.8	2.8
IRIS+ CILIARY BODY	2.0	3.0	1.1
AQUEOUS HUMOR	1.9	9.4	4.6

50 μl of 7-^{14}C-labeled drug solutions were applied to the rabbit cornea and lids closed for 30 seconds.
* The ratio was calculated from the percentage of the dose as epinephrine in the various tissues.

7. TOPICAL OPHTHALMIC CARBONIC ANHYDRASE INHIBITORS

Systemically administered carbonic anhydrase inhibitors (CAIs) such as acetazolamide, methazolamide or dichlorphenamide are known to lower intraocular pressure in glaucoma patients (Becker, 1954, Maren, 1967, Friedland & Maren, 1984). The topical instillation of these compounds has never been found efficacious.

To try and demonstrate a reduction of IOP, various formulations have been used in the topical application of CAIs. In the rabbit, for example, dichlorphenamide had to be administered as a 10% solution, 50 μl, as its sodium salt (Lotti et al, 1984b). Trifluoromethazolamide, on the other hand, significantly decreased IOP after five drops of a 2.5% suspension (Stein et al, 1983). Topical activity has also been demonstrated by Friedman et al, (1985) when soft contact lens were soaked in alkalinized solutions of acetazolamide and methazolamide.

The repeated failure of attempts to show activity after topical administration of these drugs to patients can be related to poor ocular penetration (Stein *et al*, 1983, de Feo *et al*, 1975). Considering some key physico-chemical properties of some of these compounds, it can be noticed some did not have optimal water and lipid solubilities. From the studies of Schwam *et al* (1984), Eller *et al* (1985) and Maren & Jankowska (1985), it is possible to tabulate some key properties :

Table 3

COMPOUND	pK_A	AQUEOUS SOLUBILITY (pH OF BUFFER) mg/ml	PARTITION* COEFFICIENT
Acetazolamide	7.2	2.2 (7.8)	0.001
Methazolamide	7.3	5.9 (7.8)	
Trifluormethazolamide	6.6	35 (7.8)	
Dichlorphenamide	8.3/9.8	0.7 (7.8)	
Ethoxzolamide	8.12	0.015 (7.8)	30
6-Hydroxyethoxzolamide	7.88	0.31 (7.65)	
6-Aminozolamide	8.03	0.27 (7.65)	
L-645,151	7.75	0.03 (7.0)	157
L-643,799	7.81/9.26	0.7 (6.5)	0.008

* Chloroform / pH 7.4 McIlvaine buffer at 33°C.

A typical example of an oral CAI is acetazolamide. Its poor solubility at neutral pH, together with a low partition coefficient into the lipid phase does not favor good transcorneal penetration. The ideal properties of a topically active carbonic anhydrase inhibitor have been defined by Maren (U.S. patent 729,907) :- (a) pK_a of not greater than 7.0; (b) ether partition coefficient of at least 1.0; (c) chloroform partition coefficient of at least 0.01, (d) dissociation constant against carbonic anhydrase of not more than 3×10^{-8}M; (e) first order rate constant of the penetration of the CAI through a rabbit cornea of at least 0.0002 hr^{-1}; (f) not injurious to the cornea; and (g) stable in solution and in contact with the cornea. He also claimed that if 99%+ of the enzymatic activity has to be inhibited to obtain a significant decrease of the aqueous humor secretion (Maren, *et al*, 1983), it is therefore understandable that a critical concentration of a drug must be attained in the ciliary process, the site of action to affect IOP.

Since topical efficacy is dependent on whether or not the compound crosses the cornea, a comparison of results of *in-vitro* transcorneal penetration studies for some related CAIs has been made (Table 4). Although the experiments were not performed in exactly the same way and the results are not reported in the same units, it can be noted that the ranking order of the compounds is the same.

Table 4

COMPOUNDS	IN-VITRO TRANSCORNEAL PENETRATION ACCORDING TO :		
	SCHWAM & AL	ELLER & AL	MAREN & JANKOWSKA
Acetazolamide	12	-	0.37
Methazolamide	-	-	1.9
Trifluormethazolamide	-	-	2.8
(6-derivative) Benzothiazole-2-sulphonamide			
EtO-(Ethoxzolamide)	253	43	40
$HOCH_2CH_2O$-(Hydroxyethoxzolamide)	-	1.48	-
HO-(L-643,799)	17	5.64	-
NH_2-(Aminozolamide)	-	6.7	-
Me_3.COCO-(L-654,151)	777	-	-

(1) Schwam et al (1984) as picomole/min/cm^2
(2) Eller et al (1985) as apparent corneal permeability (cm/s)
(3) Maren & Jankowska (1985) as $K_{in} \times 10^3 \times hr$

Examination of this and the previous table shows that the modification of L-643,799 into L-645,151 :-

L-643,799 L-645,151

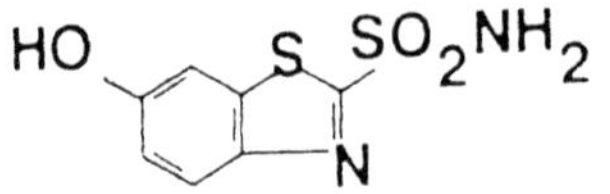

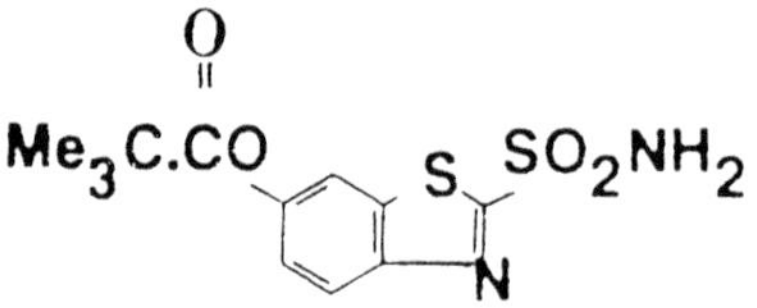

HO–(benzothiazole)–SO_2NH_2 $Me_3C.CO$–(benzothiazole)–SO_2NH_2

has considerably increased its lipophilicity, and accordingly, its transcorneal penetration. (U.S. patent 4,505,923 to Merck & Co., Schwam et al, 1984, Sugrue et al, 1985, Bar Ilan et al, 1986). Various groups (Vedani & Meyer, 1984, Eller et al, 1985, Ponticello et al, 1986, Smith et al, 1986, Jankowska et al, 1986, Maren & Jankowska, 1985, Sheppard et al, 1986) are presently investigating the structure activity relationship of analogues of ethoxzolamide and related compounds. These structural modifications of ethoxzolamide (Schoenwald et al, 1984, Schwam et al, 1984) have resulted in better transcorneal penetration and in consequence better topical activity. Thus, reduction of IOP has been reported for Carbopol™ gels of 6-hydroxyethoxzolamide (1%) by Lewis et al (1984) and 6-aminozolamide (3% in patients), Lewis et al (1986).

Efficacy has also been demonstrated for other benzothiazole-2-sulphonamides, namely the 6-hydroxy (L-643,799) and O-pivaloate (L-645,151). The elevated IOP of alpha-chymotrypsinized rabbit was significantly lowered by 0.25% suspensions of L-645,151 and 2% L-643,799 (Sugrue et al, 1985). Activity was also observed by Bar-Ilan (1986) in normal rabbits after instillation of 0.06 to 2% suspensions of L-645,151.

Ocular distribution studies after bilateral instillation of 2% suspensions, 50 µl of the compounds in the rabbit, demonstrated that only L-643,799 was found in the aqueous humor, thus indicating that the prodrug L-650,151 was quantitatively hydrolysed by corneal esterases. In addition, L-645,151 generated higher ocular concentration of L-643,799 than its parent compound. In contrast, the systemic absorption of the two CAIs was not different, as shown by the amount sequestered in the red cells :

Instillation of a 2% suspension of L-643,799

Table 5

Minutes	µg of L-643,799/gram or ml			
	Cornea	Aq Humor	Iris + C. B.	Red Cells
10	36.6 ± 11.6	0.07 ± 0.04	0.98 ± 0.70	0.99 ± 0.05
30	47.9 ± 17.2	1.03 ± 0.25	1.26 ± 0.64	2.72 ± 0.15
60	46.3 ± 16.5	2.70 ± 0.79	1.78 ± 1.59	3.48 ± 1.36
120	32.4 ± 30.7	2.48 ± 1.50	2.18 ± 0.99	5.53 ± 0.25
240	14.0 ± 11.4	1.34 ± 1.04	0.76 ± 0.62	5.41 ± 0.67

Instillation of a 2% suspension of L-645,151

Table 6

Minutes	µg of L-643,799/gram or ml			
	Cornea	Aq Humor	Iris + C. B.	Red Cells
10	101.4 ± 10.7*	0.47 ± 0.12*	1.83 ± 1.02	1.31 ± 0.20
30	91.0 ± 14.4*	3.41 ± 1.88*	4.46 ± 1.77*	2.57 ± 0.23
60	50.0 ± 28.2	3.90 ± 2.18	2.52 ± 1.02	4.30 ± 0.67
120	35.8 ± 15.5	4.28 ± 1.76	1.82 ± 0.57	4.45 ± 1.01
240	10.9 ± 8.1	1.25 ± 0.82	0.79 ± 0.68	4.80 ± 0.17

**Significantly higher ($P<0.05$) than corresponding value after instillation of L-643,799.*

Values are mean ± S.D. (N = 6) except for red cells (N = 3)

Hence, as the transcorneal penetration increases (see Table 4), the instilled amount of compound required to reduce IOP after topical application decreases. In rabbits, the progression from acetazolamide (5% in soft contact lens) through the carbopol gels of hydroxyethazolamide and aminozolamide (1%) to L-645,151 (0.2%) underlines the improvement achieved in topical CAI.

In conclusion, anti-glaucoma therapy is achieved by topical administration of compounds from many different classes of drugs. They are all however subject to the problems created by ocular fluid dynamics and trans-corneal penetration (Mikkelson, 1986).

Two approaches have been used to improve the efficacy of these drugs, namely modification of the formulation or modification of the active ingredient. Changes in formulation have been made in order to decrease the parallel pre-corneal elimination and consequently increase ocular bioavailability. Synthetic approaches have achieved a similar goal by changing the solubility (hydroxyethoxzolamide), delivering the active ingredient by means of a prodrug (L-645,151), or by increasing the lipophilicty to increase the corneal penetration.

Finally, these innovations do have drawbacks for the pharmaceutical formulation. For example, prodrugs are often esters of amides, and their facile hydrolysis often severely limits their shelf-life. Besides the difficulties of manufacturing sterile suspensions (Ashbire & Cash, 1986), the CAI sulphonamides frequently have low water solubility. This creates problems due to the saturation equilibrium existing in the formulation, for small alterations, e.g. of temperature can often lead to poor suspendability, particle growth or changes in crystal shape.

REFERENCES

Abshire R, Cash P (1986). Sterile ophthalmic ointment and suspension manufacturing. J. Parenteral Sci. and Technol. 40: 97-99

Adler CA, Maurice DM, Paterson ME (1971) The effect of viscosity of the vehicle on the penetration of fluorescein into the human eye. Exp. Eye Res. 11: 34-42

Ahmed I, Patton TF (1985) Importance of the noncorneal absorption route in topical ophthalmic drug delivery. Invest. Ophthalmol. Vis. Sci. 26: 584-587

Aldrete J, McDonald TO, De Sousa B (1983) Comparative evaluation of pilocarpine gel and timolol in patients with glaucoma. Glaucoma 5:236-241

Andermann C, Mialhe D, Arne JL, Vende D, Bec P (1983) Effet tensionnel après instillation d'une goutte de pilocarpine retard. Résultats cliniques de son action à moyen terme. J. Fr. Ophtalmol 6: 367-374

Anderson JA, Davis WL, Wei CP (1980) Site of ocular hydrolysis of a prodrug, dipivefrin, and a comparison of its ocular metabolism with that of the parent compound, epinephrine. Invest. Ophthalmol. Vis. Sci. 19: 817-823

Ariens EJ, (1974) Drug levels in the target tissue and effect. Clin. Pharmacol. Therap. 16: 155-175.

Bar-Ilan A, Pessah NI, Maren TH (1986) Ocular penetration and hypotensive activity of the topically applied carbonic anhydrase inhibitor L-645,151. J. Ocular Pharmacol. 2: 109-120

Becker B (1954) Decrease in intraocular pressure in man by a carbonic anhydrase inhibitor, Diamox. Am. J. Ophthalmol. 37: 13-15

Benedetto DA, Shah DO, Kaufman HE (1975) The instilled fluid dynamics and surface chemistry of polymers in the precorneal tear film. Invest. Ophthalmol. Vis. Sci. 14: 887-902

Benson H (1974) Permeability of the cornea to topically applied drugs. Arch. Ophthalmol. 91: 313-327

Blumenthal M, Ticho U, Zonis S, Gal A, Blank I, Mazor Z (1979) Further clinical trial with piloplex. A new long-acting pilocarpine salt. Glaucoma 1: 145

Brown RH, Hotchkiss ML, Davis EB (1985) Creating smaller eye drops by reducing eye dropper tip dimensions. Am. J. Ophthalmol. 99: 460-464

Brown RH, Lynch MG (1986) Design of eyedropper tips for topical beta-blocking agents. Amer. J. Ophthalmol. 102: 123-124

Bundgaard H, Advances in drug delivery, Churchill College, Cambridge (UK) 7-9 July 1986.

Bundgaard H, Buur A, Chang SC, Lee VHL (1986c) Prodrugs of timolol for improved ocular delivery: synthesis, hydrolysis kinetics and lipophilicity of various timolol esters. Int. J. Pharmac. 33: 15-26

Bundgaard H, Falch E, Larsen C, Mikkelson TJ (1986a) Pilocarpine prodrugs I. Synthesis, physicochemical properties and kinetics of lactonization of pilocarpic acid esters. J. Pharm. Sci. 75: 36-43

Bundgaard H, Falch E, Larsen C, Mosher GL, Mikkelson TJ (1985) Pilocarpic acid esters as novel sequentially labile pilocarpine prodrugs for improved ocular delivery. J. Med. Chem. 28: 979-981

Bundgaard H, Falch E, Larsen C, Mosher GL, Mikkelson TJ (1986b) Pilocarpine prodrugs II. Synthesis, stability, bioconversion and physicochemical properties of sequentially labile pilocarpine acid diesters. J. Pharm. Sci. 75: 775-783

Buri P, (1985) Voie oculaire. In: Buri P, Puisieux F, Doelker E, Benoît JP, (eds) Formes pharmaceutiques nouvelles, Lavoisier, Paris.

Burstein NL, Anderson JA (1985) Review: corneal penetration and ocular bioavailability of drugs. J. Ocular Pharm. 1: 309-326.

Camber O (1985) An in-vitro model for determination of drug permeability through the cornea. Acta. Pharma. Suec. 22: 335-342.

Chang SC, Bundgaard H, Lee VHL (1986b) Prodrug administration is more effective than drop size manipulation in reducing the systemic absorption of topically applied timolol in the pigmented rabbit. 1st national meeting of the Americal Assocation of pharmaceutical Scientists, Washington DC, Nov. 2-6. Pharm. Res. 3: 90S

Chang SC, Lee VHL (1986a) Vehicle factors influencing the systemic absorption of topically applied timolol in the pigmented rabbit. 1st national meeting of the American Association of Pharmaceutical Scientists, Washington DC, Nov. 2-6. Pharm. Res. 3: 86S.

Chieu TW (1978) Methods to achieve sustained drug delivery - the physical approach. In: Sustained and controlled release drug delivery systems Robinson JR, (ed), New York, Marcel Dekker 228-286

Chrai SS, Makoid MC, Erikson SP, Robinson JR (1974) Drop size and initial dosing frequency problems of topically applied ophthalmic drugs. J. Pharm. Sci. 63: 333-338

Chrai SS, Patton TF, Metha A, Robinson JR (1973) Lacrimal and instilled fluid dynamics in rabbits eyes. J. Pharm. Sci. 62: 1112-1121

Chrai SS, Robinson JR (1974) Ocular evaluation of mehtylcellulose vehicle in albino rabbits. J. Pharm. Sci. 63- 1112-1121

De Feo G, Piccinelli D, Putzolu S, Silvestrini B (1975) Effects of topically instilled drugs on intraocular pressure in rabbits. Arzneim.-Forsch (Drug Res.) 25: 806-809

De Santis LM, Schoenwald RD (1978) Lack of influence of rabbit nictitating membrane on miosis effect of pilocarpine. J. Pharm. Sci. 67: 1189-1190

Doane MG, Jensen AD, Dolhman Ch (1978) Penetration routes of topically applied eye medications. Am. J. Ophthalmol. 85: 383-386

Dunn DL, Scott BS, Dorsey ED (1981) Analysis of pilocarpine and isopilocarpine in ophthalmic solutions by normal phase high performance liquid chromatography. J. Pharm. Sci. 70: 446-449

Eller MG, Schoenwald RD, Dixson JA, Segarra T, Barfknecht CF (1985) Topical carbonic anhydrase inhibitors III: Optimization model for corneal penetration of ethoxzolamide analogues. J. Pharm. Sci. 74: 155-160

Ellis PP, Matsumura M, Rendi MA (1985) Pilocarpine concentrations in aqueous humor following single drop application I. Effect of soft contact lenses. Current Eye Res. 4: 1041-1047

Eriksen SP (1980) Physiological and formulation constraints on ocular drug bioavailability. In: Robinson JR (ed) Ophthalmic drug delivery systems (1980) 55-70. Washington DC, American Pharmaceutical Association.

File RR, Patton TF (1980) Topically Applied Pilocarpine: Human pupillary response as a function of drop size. Arch. Ophthalmol. 98: 112-115

Friedland BR, Maren TH (1984) Carbonic anhydrase : Pharmacology of inhibitors and treatment of glaucoma. In: Sears ML (ed), Pharmacology of the eye, Springer Verlag, Heidelberg,

Friedman Z, Allen RC, Raph SM (1985) Topical acetazolamide and methazolamide delivered by contact lenses. Arch. Ophthalmol. 103: 963-966

Grass GM, Robinson JR (1984) Relationship of chemical structure to corneal penetration and influence of low viscosity solution on ocular bioavailability. J. Pharm. Sci. 73: 1021-1027

Gurny R (1981b) Preliminary study of prolonged acting drug delivery system for the treatment of glaucoma. Pharm. Acta. Helv. 56: 130-132

Gurny R, Boye T, Ibrahim H (1985) Ocular therapy with nanoparticulate systems for controlled drug delivery. J. Contr. Rel. 2: 353-361

Gurny R, Peppas NA, Harrington DD, Banker GS (1981a) Development of biodegradable and injectable latices for controlled release of potent drugs. Drug Develop. Ind. Pharm. 7: 1-25

Gurny R, Taylor D (1980) Development and evaluation of a prolonged acting drug delivery system for the treatment of glaucoma In: Rubinstein MH, Proceedings of the international symposium of the British Pharmaceutical Technology Conference (London), Liverpool Solid Dosage Research Unit.

Habib FS, Attia MA, El-Shanawany SM (1985) Ocular bioavailability of pilocarpine hydrochloride in combination with physostigmine salicylate from different gel formulations. Arch. Pharm. Chem.Sci. 13: 33-38

Hamard H, Schmitt C, Plazonnet B, Le Douarec JC (1975) Etude de la pénétration oculaire de la dexaméthasone. In: Demailly P, Hamard H, Luton JP (eds) Oeil et cortisone. Masson et Cie, Paris; 33-83

Harmia T, Kreuter J, Speiser P, Boye T, Gurny R, Kubis A (1986 b) Enhancement of the myotic response of rabbits with pilocarpine-loaded polybutylcyanoacrylate nanoparticles. Int. J. Pharm. 33: 187-193

Harmia T, Speiser P, Kreuter J (1986 a) A solid colloidal drug delivery system for the eye: encapsulation of pilocarpin in nanoparticles. J. Microencaps. 3: 3-12

Harmia-Pulkkinen T, Ihantola A, Tuomi A, Kristoffersson E (1986) Nanoencapsulation of timolol by suspension and micelle polymerization. Acta Pharma. Fennica 95: 89-96

Heilman K (1984) Therapeutic systems for local use. Ocular therapeutic systems. In: Therapeutic systems (2nd ed). Stuttgart, Georg Thieme Verlag.

Holly FJ, Lemp MA (1973) The precorneal tear film and dry eye syndromes. In: Int. Ophthalmol. Clin. 13(1) Boston, Little Brown & Co.

Huang HS, Schoenwald RD, Lach JL (1983a) Corneal penetration behaviour of β-blocking agents II: Assessment of barrier contributions. J. Pharm. Sci. 72: 1272-1279

Huang HS, Schoenwald RD, Lach JL (1983b) Corneal penetration behavior of β-blocking agents III: In-Vitro - In-Vivo correlations. J. Pharm. Sci. 72: 1279-1281

Hui HW, Robinson JR (1985) Ocular delivery of progesterone using a bioadhesive polymer. Int. J. Pharm. 26: 203-213

Hui HW, Robinson JR (1986). Effect of particle dissolution rate on ocular drug bioavailability. J. Pharm. Sci. 75: 280-287.

Jankowska LM, Bar-Ilan A, Maren TH (1986) The relations between ionic and non-ionic diffusion of sulfonamides across the rabbit cornea. Invest. Ophthalmol. Vis. Sci. 27: 29-37.

Kaila T, Salminen L, Huupponen R (1985) Systemic absorption of topically applied ocular timolol. J. Ocular Pharmacol. 1: 79-83

Katz IM, Berger ET (1979) Effects of iris pigmentation on response of ocular pressure to timolol. Surv. Ophthalmol. 23: 395-398

Katz IM, Blackman WM (1977) A soluble sustained-release ophthalmic delivery unit. Am. J. Ophthalmol. 83: 728-734

Kennedy JM, McNamara PE (1981) High peformance liquid chromatographic analysis of pilocarpine hydrochloride, isopilocarpine, pilocarpic acid, and isopilocarpic acid in eye drop preparations. J. Chromatogr. 212: 331-338

Klein HZ, Miguel L, Shields MB, Leon J, Duzman E (1985) A dose-response study of piloplex for duration of action. Am. J. Ophthalmol. 99: 23-26

Krause PD (1980) Dipivefrin (DPE): Preclinical and clinical aspects of its development for use in the eye. In: Robinson JR, (ed) Ophthalmic drug delivery systems. Washington, American Pharmaceutical Association, 91-104

Kreienbaum MA, Page DP (1986) Stability of pilocarpine hydrochloride and pilocarpine nitrate ophthalmic solutions submitted by U.S. hospitals. Am. J. Hosp. Pharm. 43: 109-117

Lederer CM, Harold RE (1986) Drop size of commercial glaucoma medications. Amer. J. Ophthalmol. 101: 691-694

Lee VHL (1983) Esterase activities in adult rabbit eyes. J. Pharm. Sci. 72: 239-244

Lee VHL, Robinson JR (1982) Disposition of pilocarpine in the pigmented rabbit eye. Int. J. of Pharm. 11: 155-165.

Lee VHL, Robinson JR (1986) Review: Topical ocular drug delivery: recent developments and future challenges. J. Ocular Pharmacol. 2: 67-108

Lewis RA, Schoenwald RD, Barfknecht CF, Phelps CD (1986) Aminozolamide gel. A trial of a topical carbonic anhydrase inhibitor in ocular hypertension. Arch. Ophthalmol. 104: 842-849

Lewis RA, Schoenwald RD, Eller MG, Barfknecht CF, Phelps CD (1984) Ethoxzolamide Analogue Gel: A topical carbonic anhydrase inhibitor. Arch. Ophthalmol. 102: 1821-1824

Lotti VJ, Gautheron PD, Schmitt CJ (1984b) Topical ocular hypotensive activity and ocular penetration of dichlorphenamide sodium in rabbit. Graefe's Arch. Clin. Exp. Ophthalmol. 222: 13-19

Lotti VJ, Le Douarec JC, Stone CA (1984a) Autonomic nervous system: Adrenergic antagonists. In: Sears ML (ed) Pharmacology of the eye. Berlin-Heidelberg. Springer Verlag 248-277

Ludwig A, Van Ooteghem M (1986a) The study of the precorneal dynamics of ophthalmic solutions by fluorophotometry. Pharm. Acta. Helv. 61: 236-240

Ludwig A, Van Ooteghem M (1986b) The influence of the dropsize on the elimination of an ophthalmic solution from the precorneal area of human eyes. Drug Development Ind. Pharm. 12: 2231-2242.

Lyons JS, Krohn DL (1974) Pilocarpine uptake by pigmented uveal tissue. Am.J. Ophthalmol. 75: 883-885

Maichuk YF (1975a) Ophthalmic drug inserts. Invest. Ophthalmol. 14: 87-90

Maichuk YF (1975b) Soluble ophthalmic drug inserts. The Lancet 1: 173

Mandell AI, Stentz F, Kitabachi AE (1978) Dipivalyl epinephrine: a new prodrug in the treatment of glaucoma. Ophthalmology 85: 268-275

March WF, Stewart RM, Mandell AI, Bruce LA (1982) Duration of effect of pilocarpine gel. Am. J. Ophthalmol. 100: 1270-1271

Maren TH (1967) Carbonic anhydrase : chemistry, physiology and inhibition. Physiol. Rev. 47: 595-781

Maren TH, Jankowska L (1985) Ocular pharmacology of sulfonamides: the cornea as barrier and depot. Current Eye Res. 4: 399-408

Maren TH, Jankowska L, Sanyal G, Edelhauser HF (1983) The transcorneal permeability of sulfonamide carbonic anhydrase inhibitors and their effect on aqueous humor secretion. Exp. Eye Res. 36: 457-480.

Maren TH, Sanyal G (1983a) The activity of sulfonamides and anions against the carbonic anhydrases of animal plants and bacteria. In: George et al (eds), Annual review of pharmacology and toxicology Vol 23, Palo Alto Annual Review Inc.

Maurice DM & Mishima S (1984) Ocular pharmacokinetics. In: Sears ML (ed) Pharmacology of the eye. Vol. 69, Springer Verlag, Heidelberg, pp.19-116

McClure DA (1975) The effect of a prodrug of epinephrine (dipivaloyl epinephrine) in glaucoma - general pharmacology, toxicology and clinical experiences. In: Higuchi T, Stella V (eds): Pro-drugs as novel drug delivery systems (ACS Symposium 14) American Chemical Society, Washington D.C. pp. 224-235.

McLaughlin MA, Chiou GCY (1985) Review: a synopsis of recent developments in antiglaucoma drugs. J. Ocular Pharm. 1: 101-121.

Melis-Decerf C, Van Ooteghem M (1979) An in vitro method simulating drug release from viscous eye drops in rabbit and man. J. Pharm. Pharmacol. 31: 12-15

Mikkelson TJ (1986) Ophthalmic drug delivery. Pharm. Technol. 8: 90-98

Mindel JS, Smith H, Jacobs M, Kharlamb AB, Friedman AH (1984) Drug reservoirs in topical therapy. Invest. Ophthalmol. Vis. Sci. 25: 346-350.

Mishima S (1981) Clinical pharmacokinetics of the eye. Invest. Ophthalmol. Vis. Sci. 21: 504-541

Mishima S, Gasset A, Klyce SD Jr, Baum JL (1966) Determination of tear volume and tear flow. Invest. Ophthalmol. 5: 264-276

Mitra AK, Mikkelson TJ (1982) Ophthalmic solution buffer systems I. the effect of buffer concentration on the ocular absorption of pilocarpine. Int. J. Pharm. 10: 219-229

Noordham A, Maat L, Beyerman HC (1981) Quantitative determination of pilocarpine, isopilocarpine, pilocarpine acid and isopilocarpic acid in clinical ophthalmic pilocarpine formulations by reverse phase liquid chromatography. J. Pharm. Sci. 70: 96-97

Olijnik O, Stevens J, Wilson CG, Hardy J (1985) Ocular retention of ophthalmic vehicles evaluated in the rabbit by gamma scintigraphy. J. Pharm. Pharmacol. 37: suppl. 118P

Ono S, Hirano H, Obaka K (1971) Degradation in the side chain of cortisol by lens homogenate. Tohoku J. Exp. Med. 104: 171-175

Park K, Robinson JR (1982) Polymer binding to epithelial cells. In: Bundgaard H, Bagger Hansen A, Kofod H (eds) Optimization of drug delivery (Alfred Benzon Symposium 17) Copenhagen 1982,Munksgaard 35-49

Patton TF (1977) Pharmacokinetic evidence for improved ophthalmic drug delivery by reduction of instilled volume. J. Pharm. Sci. 66: 1058-1059

Patton TF, Ocular Drug Disposition In: Ophthalmic Drug Delivery Systems, Robinson JR, (ed), American Pharmaceutical Association, Washington D.C. 1980 pp. 28-54.

Patton TF, Robinson JR (1975) Ocular evaluation of polyvinyl alcohol vehicle in rabbits. J. Pharm. Sci. 64: 1312-1316

Patton TF, Robinson JR (1976) Quantitative precorneal disposition of topically applied pilocarpine. J. Pharm. Sci. 65: 1295-1301

Plazonnet B, Cerdeno A (1976). In-vivo hydrolysis of pilocarpine in the rabbit presented at the 5th European Workshop on Drug Metabolism, Stockholm, June 14-18.

Podos SM, Becker B, Assef C, Hartstein J (1972) Pilocarpine therapy with soft contact lenses. Am. J. Ophthalmol. 73: 336-341

Ponticello GS, Schwam H, Sugrue MF, Baldwin JJ (1986) Thienothiopyran-2-sulfonamides: Topically effective water soluble carbonic anhydrase inhibitors. 192nd ACS National Meeting, Anaheim, CA. Sept 7-12.

Prince JH (ed) (1964) The rabbit in eye research. Thomas, Springfield

Robert C, Buri P (1986) Le mucus et son rôle dans l'absorption des médicaments. Pharm. Acta. Helv. 61: 210-214

Robinson JR, Li VHK (1984) Ocular disposition and bioavailability of pilocarpine from Piloplex and other sustained drug delivery systems. In: Ticho U, and David R, (eds) Recent Advances in Glaucoma. Amsterdam, Elsevier; pp.231-236

Saettone MF, Giannaccini B, Barattini F, Tellini N (1982) The validity of rabbits for investigations on ophthalmic vehicles: a comparison of four different vehicles containing tropicamide in humans and rabbits. Pharm. Acta. Helv. 57: 47-55

Saettone MF, Giannaccini B, Chetoni P, Galle G, Chiellini E (1984b) Vehicle effect in ophthalmic bioavailability : an evaluation of polymeric inserts containing pilocarpine. J. Pharm. Pharmacol. 36: 229-234.

Saettone MF, Giannaccini B, Guiducci A, Savigni P (1986) Semisolid ophthalmic vehicles. III. An evaluation of four organic hydrogels containing pilocarpine. Int. J. of Pharma. 31: 261-270.

Saettone MF, Giannaccini B, Ravecca S, La Marca F, Tota G (1984a) Polymer effects on ocular bioavailability - the influence of different liquid vehicles on the mydriatic response of tropicamide in humans and in rabbits. Int. J. of Pharm. 20: 187-202.

Saettone MF, Giannaccini B, Savigni P, Teneggi A (1981) Vehicle effects on ophthalmic bioavailability: the influence of various vehicles on the activity of pilocarpine of rabbit and man. In: Aiäche JM, 1st European Congress of Biopharmacy and Pharmacokinetics, Clermont Ferrand, Vol 1 pp 151-155.

Saettone MF, Giannaccini B, Teneggi A, Savigni P, Tellini N (1982) Vehicle effects on ophthalmic bioavailability : the influence of different polymers on the activity of pilocarpine in rabbit and man. J. Pharm. Pharmacol. 34: 464-466

Schoenwald RD, Huang HS (1983) Corneal penetration behaviour of B-blocking agents I: Physicochemical factors. J. Pharm. Sci. 72: 1266-1272

Schoenwald RD, Ward RL, De Santis LM, Roehrs R.E. (1978) Influence of high-viscosity vehicles on miotic effect of pilocarpine. J. Pharm. Sci. 67: 1280-1283

Schwam H, Michelson SR, Sondy JM, Smith RL (1984) L-645,151 a topically effective ocular hypotensive carbonic anhydrase inhibitor: Part I, Biochemistry and metabolism. Invest.Ophthalmol. 25 (suppl): 181

Sears ML (ed) (1981) New directions in ophthalmic research. New Haven, Yale University Press

Shell JW (1982) Ocular drug delivery systems - a review. J. Toxicol.-Cut.& Ocular Toxicol. 1: 49-63

Shell JW (1984) Ophthalmic drug delivery systems. Surv. Ophthalmol. 29: 117-128

Shell JW, Baker RW (1974) Diffusional systems for controlled release of drugs to the eye. Ann. Ophthalmol. 6: 1037

Sheppard KL, Anderson PS, Graham SL, Schwam H, Smith RL, Sugrue MF (1986) Benzo[b] thiophene-, benzo[b] furan and indole-2 sulfonamides : new classes of topically effective carbonic anhydrase inhibitors. Presented at the 192nd American Chemical Society meeting, Anaheim, Ca. Sept. 7-12

Sieg JW, Robinson JR (1975) Vehicle effects on ocular bioavailability.1. Evaluation of fluorometholone. J. Pharm. Sci. 64: 931-936

Sieg JW, Triplett JW (1980) Precorneal retention of topically instilled micronized particles. J. Pharm. Sci. 69: 863-864

Smith RL, Anderson PS, Bicking JB, de Solms J, Graham SL, Hoffman JM, Michelson SR, Robb CM, Schwam H, Shepard KL, Smith AM, Scholz TH, Sondey JM, Strohmaler KM, Woltersdorf OW Jr (1986) Topical carbonic inhibitor design. Presented at the 22èmes Rencontres Internationales de Chimie Thérapeutique, Clermont Ferrand (France) Sept. 3-5

Stein A, Pinke R, Krupin T, Glabb E, Podos SM, Serle J, Maren TH (1983) The effect of topically administered carbonic anhydrase inhibitors on aqueous humor dynamics in rabbits. Am. J. Ophthalmol. 95: 222-228.

Sugaya M, Nagataki S (1978) Kinetics of topical pilocarpine in the human eye. Japan J. Ophthalmol. 22: 127-141

Sugrue MF, Gautheron P, Schmitt C, Viader MP, Conquet P, Smith RL, Share NN, Stone CA (1985) On the pharmacology of L-645,151: A topically effective ocular hypotensive carbonic anhydrase inhibitor. J. Pharmacol. Exp. Therapeutics 232: 534-540

Ticho U, Blumenthal M, Zonis S, Gal A, Blank I, Mazor Z (1979a) A clinical trial with piloplex. A new long-acting pilocarpine compound. Preliminary report. Ann. Ophthalmol. 11: 555-561

Ticho U, Blumenthal M, Zonis S, Gal A, Blank I, Mazor Z (1979b) Piloplex, a new long-acting pilocarpine polymer salt. A. Long-term study. Br.J. Ophthalmol 63: 45-47

Urbanyi T, Piedmont A, Willis E (1976) Simultaneous determination of pilocarpine and isopilocarpine in pharmaceutical preparations by liquid chromatography. J. Pharm. Sci. 65: 257-260

Urquhart J, (1980) Development of the OCUSERT® pilocarpine ocular therapeutic systems - a case history in ophthalmic product development In: Ophthalmic Drug Delivery Systems, Robinson JR, (ed), American Pharmaceutical Association, Washington D.C. pp. 105-118

Urtti A (1985) Pilocarpine release from matrices of alkyl half-esters of poly(vinyl methyl ether/maleic anhydride). Int. J. Pharm. 26: 45-55

Urtti A, Juslin M, Miinalainen O (1985a) Pilocarpine release from hydroxypropyl-cellulose-polyvinylpyrrolidone matrices. Int. J. Pharm. 25: 165-178

Urtti A, Salminen L, Miinalainen O (1985b) Systemic absorption of ocular pilocarpine is modified by polymer matrices. Int. J. Pharm. 23: 147-161

Vadnere M, Amidon G, Lindenbaum S, Haslam JL (1984) Thermodynamic studies on the gel-sol transition of some pluronic polyols. Int. J. Pharm. 22: 207-218

Van Ooteghem M (1983) Viskosität. In: Dolder R, Skinner FS (eds) Ophthalmika, Stuttgart. Wissenschaftliche Verlagsgesellschaft 372-384

Vareilles P, Schmitt C, Lotti VJ, Le Douarec JC (1978) Etude expérimentale du timolol: un nouvel hypotenseur oculaire. J. Fr. Ophtalmol. 12: 717-721

Vareilles P, Silverstone D, Plazonnet B, Le Douarec JC, Sears ML, Stone CA (1977) Comparison of the effects of timolol and other adrenergic agents on intraocular pressure in the rabbit. Invest. Ophthalmol. Vis. Sci. 16: 987-996

Vedani A, Meyer EF (1984) Structure-activity relationships of sulfonamide drugs and human carbonic anhydrase C: Modeling of inhibitor molecules into the receptor site of the enzyme with an interactive computer graphics display. J. Pharm. Sci. 73: 352-358

Waltman SR, Kaufman HE (1970) Use of hydrophilic contact lenses to increase ocular penetration of topical drugs. Invest. Ophthalmol. 9: 250-255

Wei CP, Anderson JA, Leopold I (1978) Ocular absorption and metabolism of topically applied epinephrine and a dipivalyl ester of epinephrine. Invest. Ophthalmol. Vis. Sci. 17: 315-321.

Wilson CG, Olijnik O, Hardy JG (1983) Precorneal drainage of polyvinyl alcohol solutions in the rabbit assessed by gamma scintigraphy. J. Pharm. Pharmacol. 35: 451-454.

Wood RW, Li VHK, Kreuter J, Robinson JR (1985) Ocular disposition of poly-hexyl-2-cyano 3-^{14}C acrylate nanoparticles in the albino rabbit. Int. J. Pharm. 23: 175-183

Yakovlev AA, Lenkevich MM (1966) Use of pilocarpine impregnated alcohol films in the treatment of glaucomatous patients. Vestn. Oftal. 79:40-42

Zaki I, Fitzgerald P, Hardy JG, Wilson CG (1986) A comparison on the effect of viscosity on the precorneal residence of solutions in rabbit and man. J. Pharm. Pharmacol. 38: 463-466

Zimmermann TJ, Kaufman HE (1977) Timolol: a B-adrenergic blocking agent for the treatment of glaucoma. Arch. Ophthalmol. 95: 601-604

SCINTIGRAPHIC EVALUATION OF POLYMERIC FORMULATIONS FOR OPHTHALMIC USE

C.G. Wilson

Department of Physiology and Pharmacology, Medical School
Queen's Medical Centre, Nottingham NG7 2UH, England

The appreciation of the behaviour of ophthalmic dosage forms *in vivo* has been limited by the lack of suitable quantitative methods. Tear sampling significantly alters the kinetics of the system because of the small volume of the tear film. The technique of gamma scintigraphy has superceded x-ray studies in the investigation of restriction of the nasolacrimal duct. It is a small step from this routine clinical application to apply the technique to the study of the precorneal behaviour of suitable markers incorporated into ophthalmic formulations. The method is associated with a low radiation dosimetry and can be safely used in man. This affords the opportunity to conduct comparative studies of the behaviour of polymeric formulations in man with established animal models such as the rabbit.

In the past, the most widely used technique to measure the disappearance of a drug from the precorneal area was by the removal of small volumes of the tear film for pharmacokinetic sampling. The volume of the normal tear film in man is estimated to approximately 7 ul, (Shell, 1982), with a tear turnover of 1.2 ul min $^{-1}$ (Mishima et al., 1966). Thus the removal of volumes even as low as 1 ul significantly perturbs the dynamics of the system. Furthermore, contact of the sampling capillary tube with the eye causes reflex blinking and increased tear flow, leading to dilution and an increase in the apparent rate of drainage.

A direct method of assessing the relative efficacy of formulations is the measurement of the pharmacodynamic response. This method has been used successfully to compare various pilocarpine formulations (Davies et al., 1977). However, the pharmacological response and the time course of drug action is influenced by many competing processes as summarised in Figure 1, and the relative importance of these factors cannot be measured by this method.

Subtle modifications to the formulation have the potential for a marked change in the response of the subject to the drug: the incorporation of adjuvants such as preservative surfactants may significantly increase drug permeation and residence. The adjuvants may themselves persist in the eye for a considerable period of time, for example the cationic surfactant, benzalkonium chloride administered at a dose of 0.01% w/v has been detected in ocular tissues nine days after administration (Edelhauser and Champeau 1984).

It is clear that the primary determinant of efficacy is the time for which the drug remains in contact with the eye. Thus an increase in ocular residence maximises the time available for action and decreases the potential for

Ophthalmic Drug Delivery. Biopharmaceutical, Technological and Clinical Aspects.
M.S. Saettone, G. Bucci, P. Speiser (eds.) Fidia Research Series, vol. 11, Liviana Press, Padova © 1987

systemic effects. A more efficacious preparation would have the advantage of less frequent application and increased patient compliance. This has been appreciated by many formulators and the incorporation of drugs into viscous bases such as petrolatum mineral - oil or 'Plastibase' to obtain a prolonged effect is a common strategy.

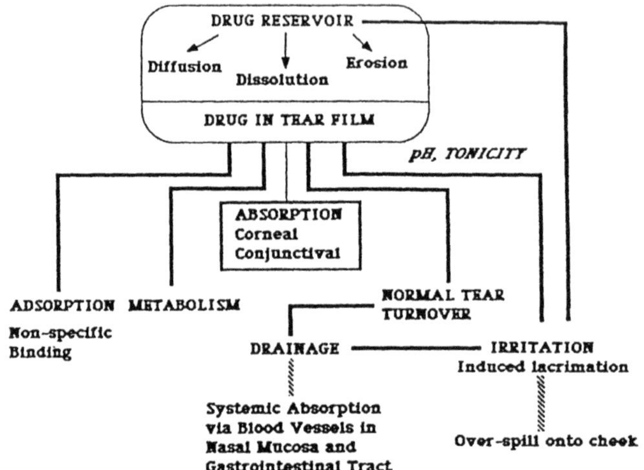

Figure 1. Summary of the processes contributing to drug absorption and loss.

However, the limitations of petrolatum - mineral oil bases, *viz.* interference with vision and gumming of the eyelids, is a serious drawback to patient acceptability. Research has, therefore, concentrated on alternative means of drug delivery using polymers, particulates and lamellar devices to obtain improved therapeutic response whilst achieving high patient tolerability. Such systems are difficult to model *in vitro*, and the high cost of animal screening programs reduces the rate of progress. Moreover, for drugs without a conveniently observable effect, for example antiviral agents, measurement of drug concentrations in the tear film provides the only opportunity to describe the kinetics of precorneal distribution.

SCINTIGRAPHIC ASSESSMENT

A non - invasive technique based on a gamma probe to measure the residence time of ophthalmic formulations labelled with technetium-99m (^{99m}Tc) was first described in 1973 by Chrai and co-workers. An important limitation of this technique is that it is not possible to resolve the distribution of activity within the eye. However, the introduction of gamma scintigraphy has largely solved this problem. The gamma camera has a large field of view, which can be split up into a matrix equivalent to several thousand finely collimated probes, making possible detailed measurements over the ocular surface and nasolacrimal duct.

The principle of operation may be described with reference to Figure 2. The pinhole collimator is used to magnify the image of the eye to allow the acquisition of more detailed information. The radiolabelled formulation is placed into the eye and the subject is positioned 5 cm from the aperture. On passing through the collimator, the gamma rays form an inverted image on a 40 cm diameter thallium-doped sodium iodide crystal. The gamma rays cause the emission of photons within the crystal and a hexagonal array of 37 photomultipliers mounted behind the crystal convert the light emitted into electrical signals giving the x and y co-ordinates of the emission. The photomultiplier signal amplitude is related to the energy of the detected gamma photon, thus the photons from different isotopes can be distinguished. Information concerning distribution of the energy is stored as a 64 x 64 pixel matrix on a minicomputer for later analysis.

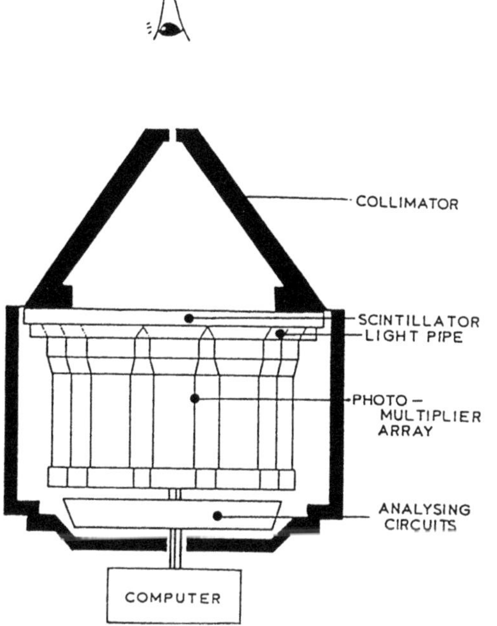

Figure 2. Schematic of construction of a gamma camera with pin-hole collimator

The diameter of the aperture of the collimator alters the resolution, whilst the distance of the source from the aperture changes the magnification. A disadvantage of the technique is that the sensitivity of the object plane is not uniform with a decrease in sensitivity occurring towards the edge of the field of view. A typical curve for a cobalt-57 flood source is shown in Figure 3. It can be seen that provided that the area of interest is kept within the central 50% of the field of view, the edge error is kept to less than 10% .

An important advantage for the pharmacokineticist is that the field of view can be arbitarily divided up into areas and the movement of isotope within these areas can be accurately followed. From such studies, it has been demonstrated that the movement of material is complex with retrograde flow (reflux) of material in the nasolacrimal duct. The division of an image into regions of interest is illustrated in Figure 4.

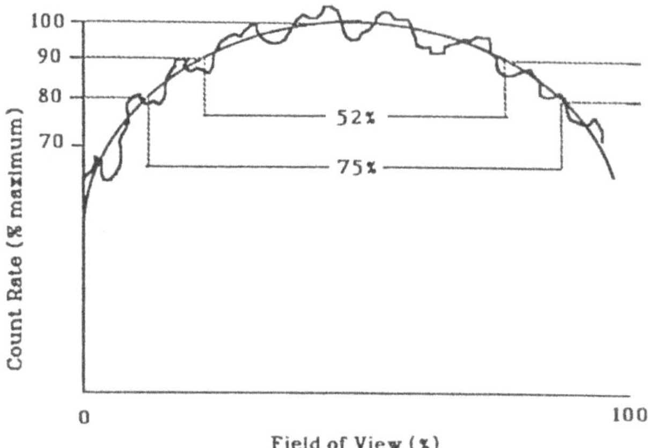

Figure 3. Uniformity of field of view assessed with gamma camera with a pin-hole collimator.

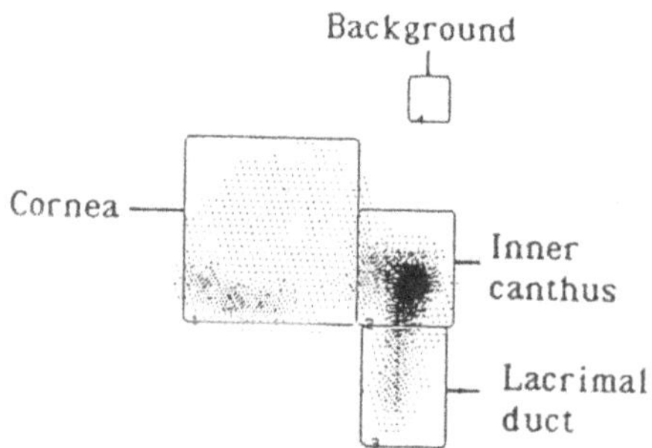

Figure 4. Division of the summed scintigraphic image into regions of interest.

CHOICE OF LABELS

The only suitable radioisotopes of carbon, nitrogen and oxygen, the usual atoms which make up substances of pharmaceutical interest, are positron emitters with very short half lives (less than 0.5 hours) and hence cannot be used for gamma imaging. The availability of suitable gamma emitting nuclides and their chemistry places severe restrictions on their use as drug labels and considerable ingenuity is needed in the design of experiments and the selection of the tracer substances. For most ophthalmic studies, non-absorbed, water-soluble markers are incorporated into the formulation dosage form in solution, e.g. Tc-99m labelled diethylenetriaminepentaacetic acid (^{99m}Tc DTPA), although lipid-soluble complexes such as indium-111 oxine can be formulated in colloidal dosage forms (nanoparticles and liposomes).

Overviews of the applications of the technique have been reviewed by Hardy and Wilson (1981) and the proceedings of a conference on the applications of gamma scintigraphy for the assessment of pharmaceutical formulations published recently (Wilson et al., 1984). In collaboration with research workers in Europe and the USA, the group at Nottingham have conducted a number of investigations into the fate of radiolabelled dosage forms in man and in rabbit. The methodology and results obtained will now be briefly reviewed.

VISCOSITY ENHANCERS

The use of viscosity enhancers such as hydroxypropyl methylcellulose (HPMC) and polyvinyl alcohol (PVA) is a common strategy to increase corneal residence time. Previously reported work by our group has demonstrated that the incorporation of 5% w/v PVA significantly increases the retention time of the radioactive marker [^{99m}Tc] sodium pertechnetate, in the rabbit eye (Wilson et al., 1983). However, the blink rate and tear turn-over time is much slower in the rabbit which suggests that this species might be less sensitive than man to the effects of solution viscosity. A comparison of HPMC and PVA solutions in the viscosity range 10.2 to 102 mPas in man and rabbit showed that solution drainage was faster in man than the rabbit with a more pronounced effect of viscosity (Zaki et al., 1986). However the overall conclusion was that the improvement, in terms of increased contact time with the cornea, was small and sustained drug delivery could not be achieved at a convenient polymer concentration.

LIPOSOMES & NANOPARTICLES

The biocompatability of liposomal formulations, and the wide interest in their application in drug targeting, encouraged workers to investigate whether these formulations were therapeutically advantageous in ophthalmic delivery. Stratford (1983) demonstrated a ten-fold increase in the ocular permeability to inulin when the marker was presented in a liposomal formulation. This was attributed to physical adsorption of liposomes onto conjunctival and corneal surfaces, followed by partitioning of the inulin into the ocular tissues. Charge and size of the liposome in the preparation has been demonstrated to be important. Schaeffer and Krohn (1982) demonstrated a greater penetration of penicillin in an *in vitro* preparation when the drug was presented in positively charged multilamellar vesicles compared to negatively charged or neutral liposomes; moreover, positively charged small unilamellar vesicles were more effective than multilamellar vesicles.

In our studies, small unilamellar vesicles have been prepared from natural lipids mixtures (egg lecithin) and synthetic lipids (dipalmitoyl-phosphatidylcholine) using the methods described by Bangham et al., (1965). The molar ratios of lipid and other constituents used to make liposomes from natural unpurified egg lecithin were as follows: egg lecithin / cholesterol / stearylamine (5:2:1) for positively charged liposomes, egg lecithin / cholesterol (9:1) for neutral liposomes, and egg lecithin / cholesterol / dicetylphosphate (5:2:1) for negative liposomes. Labelling of the liposomes with indium-111 was carried out using an adaptation of the method of

Hwang (1982) as described by Fitzgerald (1985). Labelling efficiency was between 55 and 84% according to the type of preparation and samples contained between 1 - 2 MBq in 25 ul dose. Solutions of the marker (indium-111 labelled 8-hydroxyquinoline) and technetium-99m labelled diethylenetriamine- pentaacetic acid were also tested to examine the behaviour of the label.

Six New Zealand White (NZW) rabbits were used to test each formulation. The preparation was instilled into each eye with the animal positioned in front of the gamma camera. After instillation a series of images were accumulated at 15 second intervals for a period of ten minutes and stored on the computer for later analysis. Positively charged liposomes drained more slowly than neutral or negatively charged preparations and all liposomal preparations drained more slowly than suspending buffers or solutions of the isotopes. A typical set of data obtained from the study are shown in Figure 5.

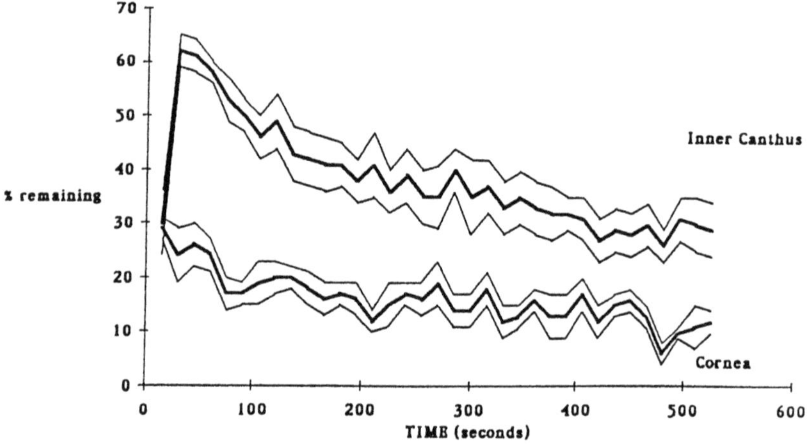

Figure 5. Kinetics of positively-charged small unilamellar vesicles in the cornea and inner canthus of the rabbit eye.

In association with Professor Kreuter's group at Zurich and Frankfurt (Fitzgerald et al., 1984), we have investigated the behaviour of radiolabelled nanoparticles, formed by anionic polymerisation of polybutyl-cyanoacrylate and labelled with indium-111 oxine. After instillation, the distribution in the cornea and inner canthus was measured (Figure 6). All particle systems tend to agglomerate and form a plug at the inner canthus and the usefulness of such systems for enhancing corneal penetration is questionable.

In the early 1980s, researchers developed two new formulation principles (Gurny 1985). Firstly, the use of vehicles with sol-gel transition temperatures in the range of 25 to 35°C and secondly pH-sensitive polymeric dispersions in the nanometer size range. These systems have been evaluated by gamma scintigraphy in collaboration with Dr Gurny (University of Geneva).

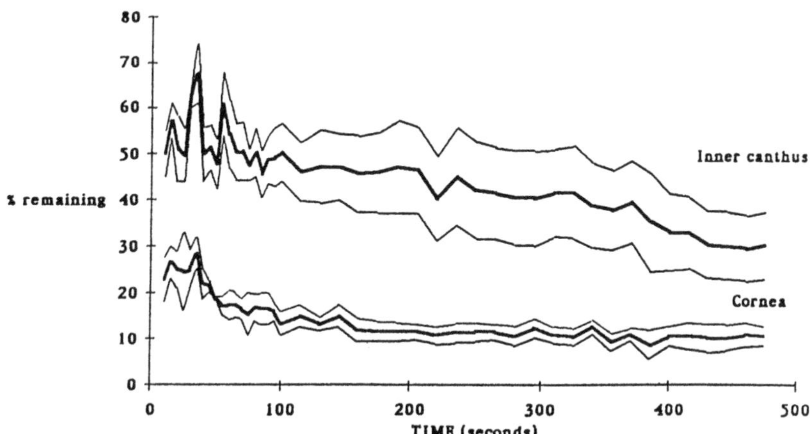

Figure 6. Distribution of nanoparticles in the cornea and inner canthus of the rabbit eye.

pH - SENSITIVE LATEX & TEMPERATURE SENSITIVE GELS.
The concept of producing a gel *in situ* in the eye has many obvious advantages which until the introduction of highly concentrated latex systems could only be achieved with inserts. A method of production of a pH sensitive nanoparticulate (latex) system has been recently described by Gurny and co-workers (1985). The method involves the emulsification of an organic solution of a suitable polymer such as cellulose acetate hydrogen phthalate (CAP) in an aqueous solution of surfactant, followed by removal of the solvent and some of the water. Drug is then added and adsorbed onto the surface of the latex nanoparticles. CAP has potentially useful properties for sustained drug delivery in the eye since the latex is a free-running solution at pH 4.4 and a gel at 7.2. Thus when placed into the eye, the pH change due to neutralization by the tear film causes an almost instant gelation of the latex. The latex particles cannot be washed out of the eye and the viscosity change reduces the rate of drainage of the aqueous phase.

An alternative stategy for achieving sustained drug delivery to the eye is to use a polymer which undergoes sol-gel transition at the temperature of the eye (33-34°C.). A suitable example is the block copolymer Pluronic F127, consisting of linked polyoxyethylene and polyoxypropylene units.

In a recent study, a 1 ml volume of the dispersion of the pseudolatex or solution of the Pluronic F127, each containing 4% pilocarpine chlorhydrate in water (as supplied by Dr Gurny), was radiolabelled by the addition of 75ul Tc-99m DTPA. These materials were compared with a solution containing 4% pilocarpine chlorhydrate in water. At the time of administration, each 25ul dose contained approximately 2 MBq. The materials were then instilled into the eyes of a group of NZW rabbits on three separate occasions and the precorneal residence measured as described previously. The results for the two polymers are shown in Figure 7.

PVA FILMS
The use of polymeric films for ocular delivery is mentioned in the British Pharmacopoeia (1948) where lamellae containing atropine for application

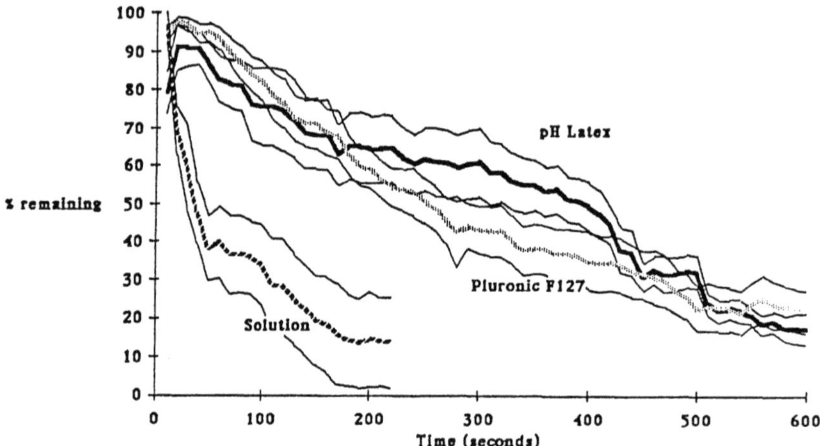

Figure 7. Drainage of ^{99m}Tc-labelled DTPA in solution, pH latex and Pluronic F127 in the rabbit.

under the lower eyelid are described. Incorporation of drugs into soluble ocular inserts formed from polyvinyl alcohol (PVA) or soluble collagen has been shown to markedly increase the penetration of drugs into the aqueous humour (Yakovlev and Lenkovich, 1966; Bloomfield et al., 1978). However, there have been few studies to measure the disposition of the soluble insert, and most measurements have been made to assess tear film concentration of the drug. The incorporation of suitable radioactive markers into a PVA film has enabled the study of the disintegration of the dosage form to be followed using gamma scintigraphy (Fitzgerald et al., 1986).

A highly soluble form of PVA (Gohsenol GH-17) was used in this study. The mean molecular weight was 98,000 with 87 - 89% hydration. 0.2 ml of ^{99m}Tc sulphur colloid, specific activity 3,500 MBq/ml, was added to 0.8 ml PVA (15 g/90 ml). This solution was then spread as a thin film, 5 mm wide by 20 cm length, onto a melinex backing sheet using a spreader with the thickness gauge set to 0.01 inches. The film was left to dry in a laminar flow cabinet and the dried film scored at 0.5 cm along its length to make 5 x 5 mm radiolabelled squares of PVA film. Immediately before use, a square was removed from the backing film. Ten healthy male and female volunteers, age range 20 - 38 years participated in the study. For the measurements, the subject was positioned at a distance of 5 cm from the collimator, with the head supported by a modified ophthalmic table. A piece of film was placed under the lower eyelid using sterile forceps. A series of images of 15 seconds duration were then acquired over a period of thirty minutes and the data stored on computer for analysis. The residence time of the film was then estimated from the scintigraphic images, with correction for background and decay rate. The data was then normalised to allow construction of the mean percentage remaining versus time for the group of ten subjects. Figure 8 shows the result obtained from the study.

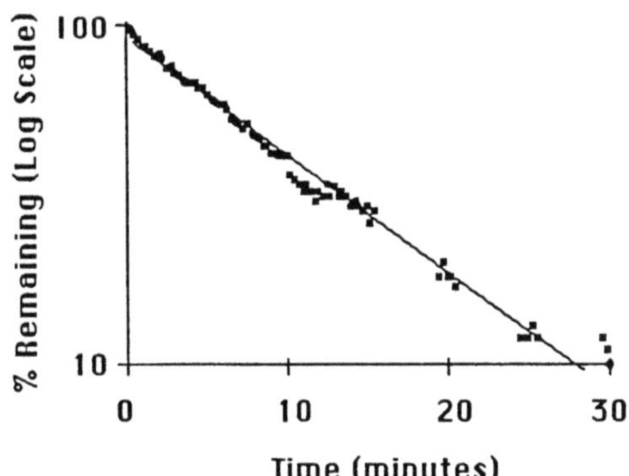

Figure 8. Mean clearance in man of ^{99m}Tc- labelled PVA film

Although there was a marked inter-individual variation in rates of dissolution, the plot of mean percentage remaining versus time follows a mono-exponential decay with a half life of around eight minutes. It is clear from these results that the PVA film remains associated with the corneal surface for a longer period than the other formulations studied. Since the amount of radioisotope incorporated into the system is very small, there is no problem in making an experimental system which includes both drug and marker. Thus it should be possible to relate the rates of dissolution within individuals to predict the variation in aqueous humour concentrations likely to be achieved in clinical practice.

Gamma scintigraphy has obvious applications in the *in vivo* assessment of ophthalmic formulations. From the limited results so far, it appears that all microparticulate formulations are swept into the corner of the eye and corneal coverage is poor. The use of sol-gel systems and film inserts would appear to have a potential which merits further investigation.

REFERENCES

Bangham A.D., Standish M.M. & Watkins J .C.(1965) J. Mol. Biol. 13: 238-252

Bloomfield S.E., Migata T., Dunn M.W. et al. (1978) Arch. Ophthalmol 96: 885-7

Chria S.S., Patton T.F., Mehta A. & Robinson J.R. (1973) J. Pharm. Sci. 62: 1112-1121.

Davies D.J.P., Jones D.E.P., Meakin B.P. & Norton D.A. (1977) Ophthalmol. Dig. 39:13-26

Edelhauser H.F. & Champeau E.J. (1984).International Tear Film Symposium Proceedings pp 47-53 (publ Lubbock:Texas)

Fitzgerald P., Hadgraft J. & Wilson C.G. (1984).J. Pharm. Pharmacol. 36: 24P.

Fitzgerald P. (1985). Ph.D. Thesis, University of Nottingham.

Fitzgerald P., Gilbert D., Hollingsbee D.A. & Wilson C. G. (1986). J. Pharm. Pharmacol (in press)

Gurny R., Boye T. & Ibrahim H. (1985) J. Control. Release. 2 : 353-61

Hardy J.G. & Wilson C.G. (1981) Clin. Phys. Physiol. Meas. 2: 71-121

Hwang K.J., Mernain J. E., Beaumier P.C. & Luk K.S.(1982). Biochimica & Biophysica Acta 716: 101-109

Mishima S., Gasset A. & Klyce S.D. (1966) Invest. Ophthalmol. 5: 264-71

Schaeffer H. E. & Krohn D.L. (1982) Invest. Ophthalmol. 23: 220-7.
Shell J.W. (1982) Surv. Ophthalmol. 26: 207-18
Stratford R.F., Yang D.C., Redell M.A. & Lee V.H.L. (1983) Int. J. Pharmaceut. 13: 263-272
Wilson C.G., Olejnik O. & Hardy J.G. (1983) J. Pharm. Pharmacol. 35: 451-4.
Wilson C.G., Hardy J. G., Frier M.& Davis S. S. eds.(1984)"Radionuclide Imaging in Formulation Research" (Croom Helm:London)
Yakovlev A.A. & Lenkovich M.M. (1966) Vestn. Oftal. 79: 40-43
Zaki, I., Fitzgerald P., Hardy J.G. & Wilson C. G. (1986) J. Pharm. Pharmac. 38: 463-466

The author gratefully acknowledges the assistance of Mrs N Washington in the preparation of this manuscript.

THE IMPORTANCE OF OPTIMIZING CORNEAL PENETRATION

R.D. Schoenwald

University of Iowa, College of Pharmacy, Iowa City, Iowa, USA

The extent of absorption occurring from the instillation of drugs topically to the eye is severely limited by physiological constraints. Consequently, it is important to consider optimizing corneal penetration in the development of a new ophthalmic drug. For some drugs an increase in the penetration rate results in a dramatic increase in effect. However, for certain drugs other pharmacokinetic processes, i.e. distribution, may be more critical to increased effectiveness. Examples are presented.

INTRODUCTION

Drug effectiveness from systemic administration depends upon the drug's intrinsic pharmacological activity as well as its pharmacokinetic properties, absorption, distribution and elimination. The pharmacologist and the medicinal chemist often collaborate to optimize the intrinsic activity of a drug. The pharmacokinetic properties of the drug are studied but only rarely are they optimized to produce a more effective drug.

Until recent years, the development of ophthalmic drugs has depended upon identifying candidates that were originally intended for systemic use. However, with the introduction of the Ocusert (Sendelbeck (1975)) and dipivefrin (Anderson, Davis and Wei (1980)), researchers in the field of ophthalmology have become aware of the potential of controlling corneal penetration for therapeutic benefit.

CLINICAL SIGNIFICANCE

Improvement in membrane penetration from increased lipophilicity has been used as a method to improve the gastrointestinal absorption of hydrophilic drugs (Notari (1976)). In particular, the penicillins, cephalosporins, tetracylines, erythromycin and lincomycin are examples that have shown improved absorption from chemical modification. The only prodrug used clinically in the eye is dipivefrin which is hydrolyzed rapidly in the cornea to epinephrine ($t_{1/2}$ = 8-10 minutes). Experiments have show that approximately 10 times more dipivefrin penetrates the eye as epinephrine when both drugs are instilled in equal doses (Anderson, Davis and Wei (1980)).

Ophthalmic drugs which have been modified into prodrugs and shown to improve corneal absorption are phenylephrine (Chien and Schoenwald (1986)), timolol (Lee and Robinson (1986)), pilocarpine (Bundgaard et al. (1985)) and nadalol (Duzman et al. (1983)). In the eye, the primary advantage from increased penetration has been the possibility of significantly reducing the instilled dose. For drugs which have the potential to cause serious systemic side effects, such as phenylephrine and timolol, the use of a prodrug would be clinically beneficial.

CORNEAL PENETRATION

Penetration across the cornea, which occurs by simple passive diffusion, is regarded as the major route by which drugs gain access into the eye. The

Ophthalmic Drug Delivery. Biopharmaceutical, Technological and Clinical Aspects.
M.S. Saettone, G. Bucci, P. Speiser (eds.) Fidia Research Series, vol. 11, Liviana Press, Padova

epithelium has been considered the major barrier to penetration across the cornea. Although corneal penetration is rapid, the tear drainage rate competes for drug so that only about 1-10% of the instilled dose is actually absorbed into the eye (Schoenwald (1985)).

Entry into the eye by scleral penetration has not been well studied and conflicting results have been published. For example, Doane et al. (1978) determined that the contribution of scleral penetration of hydrocortisone or pilocarpine into the aqueous humor or iris/ciliary body was relatively minor. However, Patton (1980) found that scleral penetration was a significant route for pilocarpine.

Anatomically, the cornea consists of five distinct layers which anterially to posterially are the epithelium, Bowman's membrane, stroma, Descemet's membrane and endothelium. The epithelium and endothelium are cellular and lipophilic. The epithelium is composed of five to six layers, whereas, the endothelium is only one cell thick. The stroma represents about 90% of the thickness of the cornea. It contains 76-80% water with the remainder consisting of collagen fibrils, which provide structural support, and mucopolysaccharides. The endothelium is responsible for maintaining the overall hydration level of the cornea which is 78% (Fatt (1978)).

Relative Layer Contribution

Huang, Schoenwald and Lach (1983) measured the permeability coefficients of a group of beta blocking agents across various layers of the cornea to determine the contribution of each layer to the total diffusional resistance.

Table 1. Barrier Resistance Across Layers of the Cornea for Various Beta Blocking Agents.

	% Resistance of Barrier			
Drug	Epithelium	Stroma	Endothelium	Log DC[a]
Lipophilic				
Penbutolol	1	46	53	2.53
bufurolol	18	50	32	2.31
bevantolol	7	44	49	2.19
propranolol	7	45	48	1.62
Slightly Lipophilic				
levbunolol	58	15	27	0.72
oxprenolol	45	21	34	0.69
metaprolol	48	18	34	0.28
timolol	68	9	23	0.34
cyclophosphamide	72	10	13	0.38
Hydrophilic				
acebutolol	91	1	8	0.20
sotalol	95	1	4	-1.25
nadolol	95	1	4	-0.82
atenolol	97.5	0.5	2	-1.52
phenylephrine	95.6	0.6	3.8	-1.00
tobramycin	95.6	0.8	3.6	<-2

[a] Octanol/buffer (pH 7.65) distribution coefficient

The reciprocal of the sum of resistances for epithelium, stroma and endothelium equaled the separately determined resistance for the intact cornea. Therefore, the cornea could be treated as three barriers in series. The total diffusional resistance (R) of the cornea can be expressed according to equation 1:

$$R_{app} = 1/(P_{app}) = R_1 + R_2 + R_3 \qquad (1)$$

where, P represents the corneal permeability coefficient and the subscripts app and 1-3 represent apparent, epithelium, stroma and endothelium, respectively. Each of the three barriers significantly contributed to diffusional resistance for drugs of intermediate lipophilicity as shown in table 1. From these results, the epithelium was the predominate rate-determining barrier for hydrophilic drugs. The endothelium provided only minimal resistance, whereas, the stroma showed negligible resistance. For the most lipophilic drugs the stroma was rate-determining.

Penetration Model Relating Partitioning to Permeability

The partition coefficient, defined as the ratio of drug concentration at equilibrium between an organic and water phase, can be useful in predicting penetration across biological membranes. One of its more attractive features, when used to predict penetration relationships from structural modifications, is that the partition coefficient of functional groups can be easily determined experimentally or, if available, taken from published tables (Hansch and Leo (1983)). In either case, it is added to the value known for the parent molecule to predict the partition coefficient of the analog or prodrug.

The total diffusional resistance (R_{app}) through the intact corneal membrane as expressed by equation 1 can be expanded according to equation 2 (Schoenwald and Huang (1983)) :

$$P_{app} = \frac{1}{R_{app}} = \frac{1}{\dfrac{h_1}{D_1(PC)_1} + \dfrac{h_2}{D_2(PC)_2} + \dfrac{h_3}{D_3(PC)_3}} \qquad (2)$$

where, h is the effective thickness of the membrane, D is the diffusion coefficient and (PC) is the biological partition coefficient. The octanol-buffer(pH 7.65) distribution coefficient (DC) can be related to PC according to equation 3:

$$\log(PC)_i = a_i \log(DC)_i + b_i \qquad (3)$$

For any corneal layer, i, a plot of $\log P_i$ versus log DC will show a linear relationship with a slope of a_i and an intercept equal to $(D_i b_i/h_i)$. By taking the antilog of equation 3 and substituting the experimentally determined DC into equation 2, an expression results which can be used to generate an expected relationship for P_{app} as a function of DC:

$$P_{app} = \frac{1}{\dfrac{h_1}{D_1 b_1 (DC)^{a_1}} + \dfrac{h_2}{D_2 b_2 (DC)^{a_2}} + \dfrac{h_3}{D_3 b_3 (DC)^{a_3}}} \qquad (4)$$

For any corneal layer, i, a plot of $\log P_i$ versus log DC will show a linear relationship with a slope of a_i and an intercept equal to $(D_i b_i/h_i)$. Figure 1 is a computer generated log-log plot of equation 4 representing the experimental parameters determined for each corneal layer.

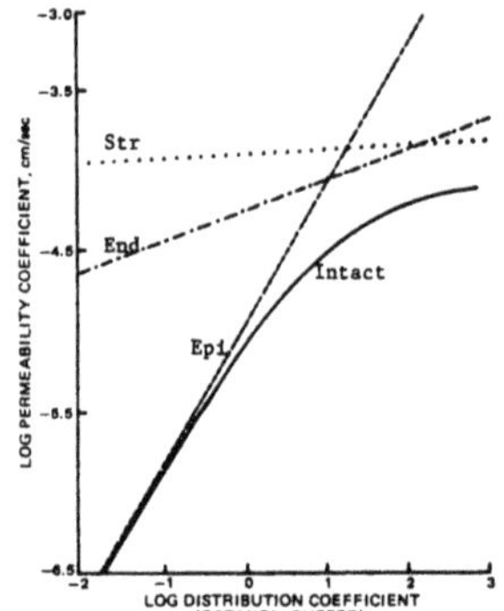

Figure 1. Computer-Generated Log-Log Plots of PC intact cornea and three separate layers versus DC (Adapted from Huang, Schoenwald and Lach (1983)).

The linear relationships in figure 1 were added to produce the curvilinear composite of the intact cornea which begins to approach a plateau between log PC 1.5 to 2.5. This occurs because of the small slope values associated with the endothelium and particularly the stroma. A similar plateau region has been identified for steroids (Schoenwald and Ward(1978)), substituted benzothiazole-2-sulfonamides (Eller et al. (1985a)) and n-alkyl-p-aminobenzoate esters (Mosher and Mikkelson (1979)).

The slope value of nearly zero for the stroma indicates that stromal permeability is independent of partitioning and that the drug is simply diffusing through the aqueous mucopolysaccharide media. This is not surprising since the stroma is non-cellular and contains 76-80% water.
The fibrils increase the diffusional path length as opposed to a linear diffusional path length through the aqueous media. A theoretical expression for R_2 can therefore be defined as follows:

$$R_2 = \frac{h_2 \ \mathrm{Tau}}{D_2 \ \mathrm{Epsilon}} \tag{5}$$

where, D_2, the diffusion coefficient in stromal fluids, equals (D_{aq}Tau)/Epsilon; Tau represents the tortuosity (dimensionless) imposed by the geometric arrangement of the collagen fibrils and Epsilon (dimensionless) represents the porosity of the stromal matrix. D_{aq} is the aqueous diffusion coefficient. Figure 2 shows a schematic arrangement of the collagen structure of the stroma.

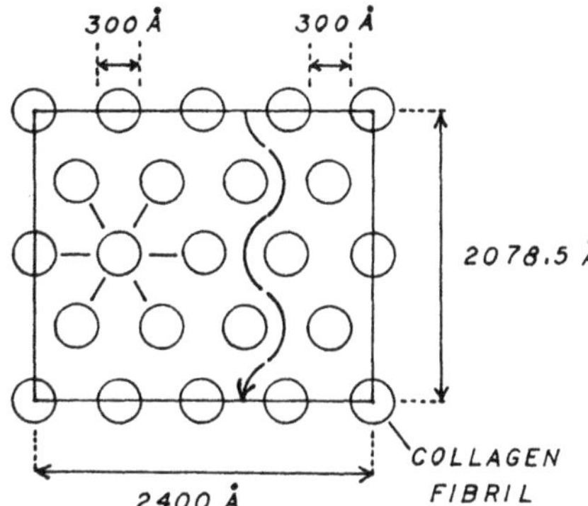

Figure 2. Arrangement of Collagen Fibrils of the Stroma. The curved arrow between the fibrils represents the diffusional pathway of least resistance. (Adapted from Huang, Schoenwald and Lach (1983)).

The collagen fibrils, 300 A in diameter, are arranged nearly parallel to one another with an open spacing of 300 A between fibrils. Based upon these dimensions, the tortuosity and porosity can be estimated as 1.21 and 0.773, respectively, resulting in a ratio of 1.56. In equation 5 both R_2 and h_2 were determined experimentally. D_{aq} could be estimated from the Sutherland-Einstein equation and the D_{aq} for benzoic acid. Consequently, a Tau/Epsilon ratio of 1.58 could be determined (Huang, Schoenwald and Lach (1983)) which agrees very closely with the estimate based upon the geometrical arrangement of the stroma shown in figure 2 (1.56).

The individual partitioning characteristics of each corneal layer, particularly the stroma, can be utilized to advantage in developing a prodrug. When optimized for penetration, a lipophilic prodrug will rapidly penetrate the epithelium. If enzymatic hydrolysis is rapid, the hydrophilic drug will accumulate in the stroma at a faster rate than penetration across the endothelium. As a result the hydrophilic drug species will be slowly released from the stroma allowing high concentrations to be maintained in the anterior chamber for a prolonged period. This phenomena may explain the prolongation of duration of diester prodrugs of pilocarpine (Bundgaard et al. (1985)).

Penetration Model Relating Structual Parameters to Permeability

Corneal penetrability can be characterized with the use of the partition coefficient. However, this approach only permits the structure of an optimally penetrating drug candidate to be defined in terms of its partitioning behavior, not its exact structure. The electronic effects of a particular substituent influence penetration, particularly through pK_a or polarity, and therefore must also be considered.

In order to more accurately define an optimally penetrating structure, Eller et al. (1985a) related structural parameters to permeability for an analog series representing modification to the benzene ring of 2-benzothiazolesulfonamide. Ethoxzolamide, a member of the series, is a carbonic anhydrase inhibitor (CAI) which is effective in lowering intraocular pressure (IOP) when taken orally by glaucoma patients but is not effective when dosed topically to the eye.

Table 2. Chemical Structure of Ethoxzolamide and Related Analogs With Substituents Added to the Benzene Ring.

Compound	Mol. Wt.	Substituent X_4	X_5	X_6	X_7
6-Hydrogen	214	H	H	H	H
6-Hydroxy	230	H	H	OH	H
6-Chloro	249	H	H	Cl	H
4,6-Dichloro	283	Cl	H	Cl	H
6-Amino	229	H	H	NH_2	H
6-Ethoxy(ethoxzolamide)	258	H	H	C_2H_5O	H
6-Nitro	259	H	H	NO_2	H
6-Hydroxyethoxy	274	H	H	$HOCH_2CH_2O$	H
6-Benzyloxy	320	H	H	$C_6H_5CH_2O$	H
6-Acetamido	271	H	H	CH_3CONH	H
7-Amino-6-ethoxy	273	H	H	C_2H_5O	NH_2
6-Dimethylamino	255	H	H	$N(CH_2)_2$	H
4,7-Dimethyl-6-amino	255	CH_2	H	NH_2	CH_2

Correlation of permeability to structural parameters begins with a definition of the penetration rate across the cornea (PR):

$$PR = (CP)(C_{tears}) \quad (6)$$

In equation 6, CP represents apparent permeability coefficient across the cornea and C_{tears} is the drug concentration in the tears. The maximum penetration rate (MPR) attainable can be expressed as:

$$MPR = (CP)(\text{tear solubility}) \quad (7)$$

When drug solubility at the pH of the tears (pH 7.65) is substituted for tear solubility and CP is determined from intact excised rabbit corneas, MPR can be used to assess relative penetrability for an analog series. Table 3 lists MPR values for the CAI analogs in table 2 synthesized for the purpose of identifying optimal penetration into the eye.

Table 3. Comparison of MPR values for Ethoxzolamide and related Analogs

Compound	S_T mcg/mL	CP cm/sec(X10^{-6})	MPR ng/cm$_2$/sec
6-Hydrogen	792.2	36.2	26.7
6-Hydroxy	1349.1	5.6	7.6
6-Chloro	156.4	42.8	6.7
4,6-Dichloro	56.0	38.8	2.2
6-Amino	269.4	6.7	1.8
6-Ethoxy(ethoxzolamide)	40.9	43.9	1.8
6-Nitro	176.0	6.6	1.2
6-Hydroxyethoxy	310.4	1.5	0.5
6-Benzyloxy	2.2	47.0	0.1
6-Acetamido	209.1	4.7	1.0
7-Amino-6-ethoxy	31.3	2.2	0.7
4,7-Dimethyl-6-amino	30.8	13.7	0.4

For this series, molecular weight and lipophilicity were the critical factors that could be controlled to promote a high MPR. Smaller analogs were more soluble, possessed intermediate lipophilicity and therefore penetrated the cornea more rapidly. This occurs because a more soluble drug which maintains lipophilicity can achieve a higher concentration gradient. Compounds which are lipophilic quite often have a high CP but low solubility. Conversely, compounds which are too hydrophilic often are very soluble and have a low CP. In either case, the net result is a low penetration rate.

Although equation 7 represents a relative measure of penetrability, it does not permit selection of a functional group that predicts optimal penetration for the analog series. Identification of such an analog was accomplished by a series of substitutions relating MPR to structural parameters, sigma$_p$ and pi, through experimentally determined physico-chemical parameter values. Sigma$_p$ and pi are mathematically defined by equations 8 and 9:

$$pK_a = \text{rho}\,(\text{sigma}_p) + (pK_a)_H \qquad (8)$$

$$\log(PC)_X = c(\text{pi})_X + \log(PC)_H \qquad (9)$$

where, rho and c are equation parameters determinied from regression analysis of the experimental data. The subscript H represents the parameter values for the 6-hydrogen substitution as compared to any other substituent X at the same molecular location. Sigma$_p$ and pi are obtained from tables of values which exist for many substituent groups (Hansch and Leo (1983)).

Two other relationships were necessary in order to relate MPR to sigma$_p$ and pi. A relationship was established between the intrinsic solubility of the analogs and their respective PC values. In addition, CP could be exponentially related to DC. In each case, equation parameters for slopes and intercepts could be determined from the experimental data and regression analysis. It was possible to algebraically interrelate MPR to sigma$_p$ and pi such that MPR became a predictor of optimal penetration across the cornea (Eller et al. 1985a,b). Figure 3 is a three dimensional plot permitting these relationships to be observed.

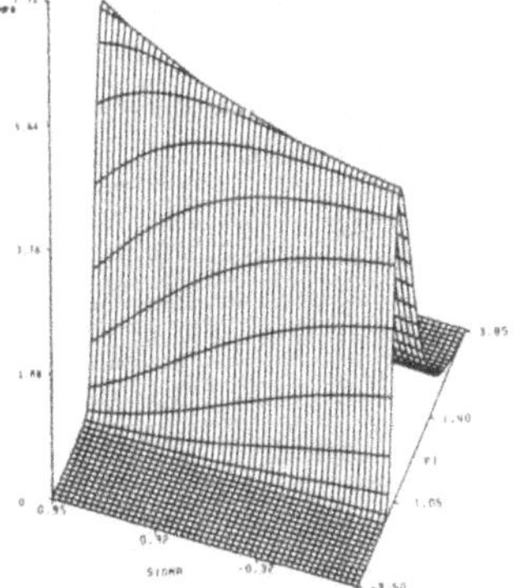

Figure 3. A three-dimensional view of the predicted MPR as a function of electronic (sigma$_p$) and lipophilic (pi) factors for 6-substituted 2-benzothiazolesulfonamides. (Adapted from Eller et al. (1985a)).

An optimal range of sigma$_p$ (-0.2 to 0.95) and pi (-0.8 to 0.1) was identified. Restraints, such as, potential toxicity of metabolic fragments, availability of a synthetic pathway and chemical stability, serve to limit the selection of an ideal analog. Nevertheless, the approach identifies an optimally penetrating compound and reduces the synthesis to a reasonably few compounds.

CONSIDERATION OF DISPOSITION PROCESSES

The 6-hydrogen analog yielded exceptionally higher MPR values than ethoxzolamide (see table 2) , and when maintained on the rabbit eye until steady state aqueous humor levels were reached, it also attained 16 fold higher steady state levels (Eller et al. (1985b). However, when instilled in the normotensive rabbit eye as a 1% gel or a 1% suspension (Eller(1984)) or as a 3% gel in the laser-induced hypertensive monkey eye (DeSantis et al.(1986)), no significant lowering of IOP was detected. Surprisingly, the 6-amino analog, which penetrated the rabbit cornea at approximately equal rates to ethoxzolamide, significantly lowered IOP in both the monkey and rabbit eye. The 6-hydroxyethoxy analog was equally active in both species yet its MPR is about 1/4 that of ethoxzolamide. More importantly, in a single dose study using a 3% gel, the 6-amino analog significantly reduced IOP in ocular hypertensive patients (Lewis et al. (1986)).

Figure 4 more clearly shows that MPR does not necessarily predict topical activity with regard to a drop in IOP for the CAI analogs. MPR values in figure 4 are relative to ethoxzolamide.

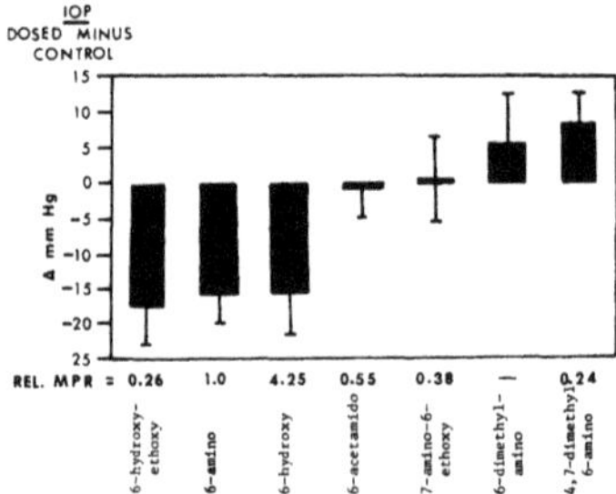

Figure 4. Effect of 3% CAI Gels on IOP in Laser-Induced Ocular Hypertensive Monkeys Seven Hours After Dosing.

Results from in vitro experiments (Putnam et al. (1986)) established that the inhibitory activity of the 6-amino analog against carbonic anhydrase B was equivalent to ethoxzolamide. Therefore, further studies were designed to investigate the ocular disposition of the 6-amino analog to explain its activity when instilled topically to the eye.

A constant concentration of 67.4 mcg/mL of drug was applied to the eye of anesthetized rabbits for 90 minutes. In addition to measuring drug, a metabolite was identified and its concentration measured from cornea, aqueous humor and iris/ciliary body. Various technics indicated that the metabolite was 6-acetamido-2-benzothiazolesulfonamide, an analog which had been previously synthesized. The metabolite did not lower IOP when dosed topically to the eye of either rabbits or monkeys. Moreover, its physico-chemical properties as well as its MPR was approximately equal to ethoxzolamide (see table 2).

Relatively high levels of the metabolite was identified in the cornea and iris/ciliary body but were 50% lower in aqueous humor. When compared to drug levels in the aqueous humor and iris/ciliary body, metabolite levels were 2 and

9-fold greater, respectively. Figure 5 graphically depicts the disposition of drug and metabolite in the rabbit eye.

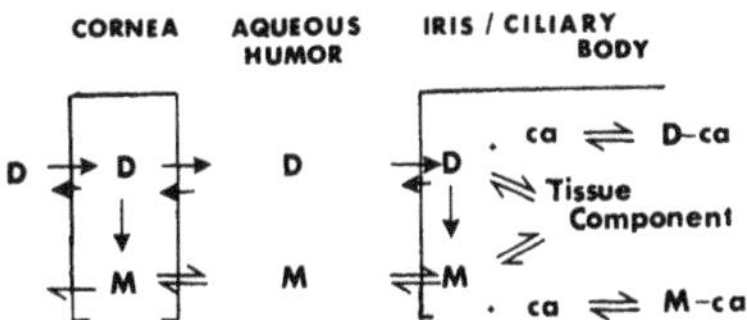

Figure 5. Graphical Representation of the Disposition of 6-amino-2-benzothiazolesulfonamide and Its Metabolite.

It is hypothesized that topical activity is a consequence of both metabolite (M) retention in the iris/ciliary body as well as inhibition of 99+ % of carbonic anhydrase (ca) by drug (D) and metabolite. Both of these events must occur over a sufficient time period to effect a significant lowering of IOP.

Although rapid corneal penetration is indeed necessary in order to achieve significant levels of drug in aqueous humor, distribution and subsequent accumulation of drug in the appropriate internal eye tissues must not be overlooked as a critical step to the therapeutic success of potential new ophthalmic drugs.

REFERENCES

Anderson JA, Davis JL and Wei CP (1980) Site of Ocular Hydrolysis of a Prodrug and a Comparison of Its Ocular Metabolism with That of the Parent Compound, Epinephrine. Invest Ophthalmol Vis Sci 19: 817-823.

Bundgaard H, Falch E, Larsen C, Mosher GL and Mikkelson TJ (1985) Pilocarpic Acid Esters as Novel Sequentially Labile Pilocarpine Prodrugs for Improved Ocular Delivery. J Med Chem 28: 979-981.

Chiang CH, Schoenwald RD (1986) Ocular Pharmacokinetic Models of Clonidine-^{3}H Hydrochloride. J Pharmacokin Biopharm 14: 175-211.

DeSantis L, Sallee V, Barnes G, Schoenwald R, Barfknecht C, Duffel M and Lewis R (1986) The Effect of Topically Applied Analogs of the Carvonic Anhydrase Inhibitor, Ethoxzolamide, on Intraocular Pressure in Alert Laser-Induced Ocular Hypertensive Cynomolgus Monkeys. Suppl to Invest Ophthalmol Vis Sci 16: 179.

Doane MG, Jensen AD and Dohlman CH (1978) Penetration Routes of Topically Applied Eye Medications. Am J Ophthalmol 85:383-386.

Duzman E, Anderson J, Vita JB, Lue JC, Chen CC and Leopold IH (1983) Topically Applied Oxymetazoline. Ocular Vasoconstrictive Activity, Pharmacokinetics, and Metabolism. Arch Ophthalmol 101: 1122-1127.

Eller MG (1984) In: Ph.D. Thesis: Optimization Model for Corneal Penetration of

Ethoxzolamide Analogs. University of Iowa, Iowa City, IA.; pp. 163-176.

Eller MG, Schoenwald RD, Dixson JA, Segarra T and Barfknecht T (1985a) Topical Carbonic Anhydrase Inhibitors III: Optimization Model for Corneal Penetration of Ethoxzolamide Analogues. J Pharm Sci 74:155-160.

Eller MG, Schoenwald RD, Dixson JA, Segarra T and Barfknecht CF (1985b) Topical Carbonic Anhydrase Inhibitors IV: Relationship Between Excised Corneal Permeability and Pharmacokinetic Factors. J Pharm Sci 74:525-529.

Fatt I (1978) Physiology of the Eye, Butterworth, Woburn Mass; pp. 114-121.

Huang HS, Schoenwald RD and Lach LL (1983) Corneal Penetration Behavior of Beta-Blocking Agents II: Assessment of Barrier Contributions. J Pharm Sci 72:1272-1278.

Hansch C and Leo A (1983) Log P and Parameter Database. Comtex Scientific Corp., New York.

Lee VHL and Robinson JR (1986) Review: Topical Ocular Drug Delivery: Recent Developments and Future Challenges. J Ocular Pharmacol 2:67-108.

Lewis RA, Schoenwald RD, Barfknecht CF and Phelps CD (1986) Aminozolamide Gel A Trial of a Topical Carbonic Anhydrase Inhibitor in Ocular Hypertension. Arch Ophthalmol 104:842-844.

Mosher GL and Mikkelson TJ (1979) Permeability of the n-alkyl-p-aminobenzoate Esters Across the Isolated Corneal Membrane of the Rabbit. Int J Pharm 2:239-243.

Notari RE (1976) Alteration of Pharmacokinetics Through Structural Modification. In: Roche EB (ed): Design of Biopharmaceutical Properties through Prodrugs and Analogs. Am Pharm Assoc Academy of Pharm Sci, Washington D.C.; 68-97.

Patton TF (1980) Ocular Drug Disposition and Pharmacokinetics. Am Pharm Assoc Academy of Pharm Sci, Abstracts 15:47.

Putnam ML, Schoenwald RD, Duffel MW, Barfknecht CF, Segarra TM and Campbell DA (1986) Ocular Disposition of Aminozolamide in the Rabbit Eye. Invest Ophthalmol Vis Sci, in press.

Schoenwald RD (1985) The Control of Drug Bioavailability from Ophthalmic Dosage Forms. In: Smolen VF and Ball LA (eds): Controlled Drug Bioavailability Volume 3: Bioavailability Control by Drug Delivery System Design. John Wiley & Sons, New York; pp. 257-306.

Schoenwald RD and Huang HS (1983) Corneal Penetration Behavior of Beta-Blocking Agents I: Physicochemical Factors. J Pharm Sci 72:1266-1272.

Schoenwald RD and Ward RL (1981) Relationship Between Steroid Permeability Across Excised Rabbit Cornea and Octanol Water Partition Coefficients. J Pharm Sci 67:786-788.

Sendelbeck L, Moore D, Urquhart J (1975) Comparative Distribution of Pilocarpine in Ocular Tissues of the Rabbit During Administration by Eye Drop or by Membrane Controlled Delivery System. Am J Ophthalmol 80: 274-283.

PILOCARPINE INSERTS: EXPERIMENTAL AND CLINICAL EXPERIENCES

L. Salminen

Department of Ophthalmology, Turku University Central Hospital
Turku, Finland

During the last 15 years about ten pilocarpine ocular inserts - most of soluble hydrophilic polymers - have been presented. In vitro studies demonstrated prolongation of pilocarpine release from these systems as compared to pilocarpine solutions. In in vivo studies in rabbits the hydrophilic inserts gelled in minutes and dissolved in hours. The magnitude of maximum pupil size constriction was enhanced, with duration of miosis significantly increased over that of liquid dosage systems. Few pilocarpine inserts have been tested in human eyes and in clinical use is only one type (Maichuk, 1976).

INTRODUCTION

An approach to extend drug residence time in the cul-de-sac, thereby prolonging drug absorption, is soluble drug inserts. Under proper conditions, the polymers used in gel formulations as well as biopolymers such as collagen and fibrin can be fabricated into erodible inserts for placement in the cul-de-sac.

Most developmental work on erodible inserts has been done with inserts delivering pilocarpine. However, also unmedicated and inserts with other ocular drugs have been presented. For the treatment of keratitis sicca unmedicated, rod and oval--shaped hydroxypropylcellulose inserts - available as a commercial preparation (Lacrisert[R] 5 mg, MSD) - (Katz and Blackman, 1977; Katz et.al., 1978) and ovoid wafers of succinylated collagen (Bloomfield et al., 1977) have been presented. In animal experiments idoxyuridine (Pavan-Langston et al., 1975), gentamycin (Bloomfield et al., 1978) and epinephrine (Birss et al., 1978) have been administered in polypeptide, succinylated collagen and polymeric matrices, respectively.

Since the introduction of sustained release pilocarpine therapy (Lerman, 1970) and the ocular insert device for continous constant-rate delivery of drugs to the eye (Dohlman et al.,1972) experimental and clinical work has been done for the development

Ophthalmic Drug Delivery. Biopharmaceutical, Technological and Clinical Aspects.
M.S. Saettone, G. Bucci, P. Speiser (eds.) Fidia Research Series, vol. 11, Liviana Press, Padova © 1987

of soluble pilocarpine inserts. Despite numerous publications on the subject, few inserts have been tested in humans and in clinical routine for the treatment of glaucoma is only one type (Maichuk, 1976, 1985; Maichuk and Erichev, 1981).

On the subject a number of excellent reviews provide background information: on ocular pharmacokinetics, ocular drug bioavailability and the recent development and future challenges of topical ocular drug delivery (Richardson, 1975; Mishima, 1981; Maurice and Mishima, 1984; Shell, 1984; Lee and Robinson, 1986).

EXPERIMENTAL EXPERIENCES WITH PILOCARPINE INSERTS

In pharmacokinetic studies pilocarpine is an ideal drug. In the eye, measurement of pilocarpine induced miosis allows a continous monitoring of pharmacological response and calculation of various pharmacokinetic parameters (Yoshida and Mishima, 1975). Albino rabbit has been the most common test animal for development and study of pilocarpine inserts. However, there is evidence that the pigmented rabbit may be a more suitable animal to use for ocular pharmacokinetic studies with pilocarpine (Salminen et al., 1984; Lee and Robinson, 1986). Even the suitability of the rabbit as an animal model to evaluate ocular drug delivery systems is limited as pointed out by Lee and Robinson, 1986. According to Saettone et al. (1982) the rabbit is less sensitive than humans to vehicle effects on ocular drug bioavailability.

During the last 15 years about ten soluble inserts of various material for ocular pilocarpine delivery have been presented. Studies of the kinetics and mechanism of pilocarpine release were made in vitro on some of them. In vivo the inserts were tested for miotic response in rabbit eyes but neither intraocular pressure determinations nor ocular tissues samples for drug concentration assay were taken.

Miotic responses to 0.075 ml of 3.34% pilocarpine alginate and 2% pilocarpine hydrochloride solutions and to pilocarpine alginate flakes (4.9 mg) were studied in albino rabbits by Loucas and Haddad (1972). The flakes were circular. The results derived from solid pilocarpine alginate deposition show the magnitude of maximum pupil size constriction to be enhanced, with duration of miosis significantly increased over that of both liquid dosage systems. Restoration of normal pupillary diameter for the solid-state dose was observed to occur between 7 and 8 h in contrast to about 3.5 h for the ophthalmic solutions.

Salminen et al. (1983) calculated apparent biophasic availability of pilocarpine in albino rabbit eyes after various doses and dosage forms. Pilocarpine doses of 0.85 and 2.30 mg in aqueous solutions, 1.00 mg in oil and 0.85 mg in a solid insert, were applied ocularly. The circular insert with a diameter of 5 mm and a thickness of 0.4 mm was a water soluble polyvinylpyrrolidone (PVP) matrix, which released 80% of its pilocarpine content in 35 min in vitro. In the inferior fornix of the eye this insert gelled in about 5 min and dissolved in 1 h. The time delay for peak pilocarpine response was 16.3-24.0 min, and the constant for apparent rate of elimination was 0.69-0.81 h^{-1}. Neither time delay nor this constant was affected by the dose and dosage form. Magnitude of the peak response and apparent biophasic availability were influenced by the vehicle and the dose:insert (0.85 mg) $>$ oily solution (1.00 mg) $>$ aqueous solution (2.30 mg) $>$ aqueous solution (0.85 mg). The insert and oily solution did not show vehicle-controlled drug absorption and can be regarded as prolonged pulse-entry medication.

The test procedure was similar as above when the time course of the miotic response of pilocarpine in albino and pigmented rabbit eyes was studied after 0.025 ml pilocarpine eye drops (0.11, 0.43, 0.85 and 2.30 mg of the drug) and after pilocarpine (0.85 and 2.30 mg) matrices of poly(acrylamide) and copolymer of acrylamide, N-vinylpyrrolidone and ethylacrylate (Urtti et al., 1984). The inserts were 4.5 mm wide, 0.35 mm thick and 3.3 mm (0.85 mg of the drug) or 9 mm (drug content 2.3 mg) long. When administered in eye drops, ocular pigmentation delayed the onset of the peak effect of the 3 smallest pilocarpine doses. The magnitude of the peak effect was lower in pigmented than in albino eyes after 0.11 and 0.43 mg doses, but equal after larger doses. Ocular pigmentation increased the relative biophasic availability of 0.85 and 2.30 mg doses of pilocarpine. This was due to the slower elimination rate of pilocarpine from pigmented tissues. The relative biophasic availability of 0.11 and 0.43 mg doses of pilocarpine were not affected by the ocular pigmentation because of the opposite effects of lower peak effect and slower elimination rate on biophasic availability in pigmented eyes. When administered in polymer matrices, pilocarpine showed a typical time course of prolonged pulse-entry of the drug into the eye.

The effects of polymeric insert properties on the miotic effect of pilocarpine have been extensively studied by Saettone et al. (1984), who used different types of soluble hydrophilic polymers: poly(vinyl alcohol) (PVA) and hydroxypropylcellulose (HPC) in their matrices. The films were 0.4-0.5 mm thick small discs, each containing 1.0 mg of pilocarpine nitrate. Although these hydrophilic matrices did not show vehicle--controlled deliver of pilocarpine in the eye, duration of miotic effect of pilocarpine was increased by decreasing the release rate of pilocarpine from the matrices.

Grass et al. (1984) delivered ocular pilocarpine from erodible matrices of polyvinyl alcohol and carboxyvinyl copolymer. In vitro studies demonstrated significant prolongation of drug release from these systems as compared with simple aqueous or viscous solutions. The in vitro results were supported by in vivo miosis studies in albino rabbits. The lamellae showed a greater miotic response and a longer period of response, as compared with the solutions.

Urtti et al. (1985a) studied the effects of hydrophilicity of polymer matrix on in vitro release rate of pilocarpine and on its miotic activity in rabbit eyes. Increasing the amount of PVP in the matrices increased the release rate and hygroscopicity of the matrices. Rod-shaped 3.2 mg matrices with 0.45 mg pilocarpine base were applied into the inferior fornix of the rabbits and the miotic effect was followed. Despite in vitro differences, the time course of miotic response did not vary between the polymer matrices. Compared to aqueous eye drop (0.025 ml of 1.8% pilocarpine), the polymer matrix administration delayed the onset of the peak effect, but did not affect its magnitude. The biophasic availability was increased 1.2-fold compared to the eye drops. The rod shape and the small size of the matrices diminished the favourable effect of polymer matrices on drug bioavailability. Administration of pilocarpine in polymer matrices probably caused conjunctival vasodilatation and subsequent systemic rather than intraocular drug absorption.

Systematic studies on the kinetics and mechanism of pilocarpine release from inserts of soluble hydrophilic polymers and of bioerodible polymers has been made by Urtti et al. (1985b) and by Urtti (1985c). The rate of release of pilocarpine was decreased by the increased molecular weight and concentration of hydroxypropylcellulose (HPC) in hydroxypropylcellulose-polyvinylpirrolidone matrices. Release of pilocarpine from hydroxypropylcellulose matrices was controlled by the diffusion of pilocarpine. Increased polymer dissolution with increased polyvinylpirrolidone concentration shifted the release profile towards dissolution-controlled kinetics.Increased molecular weight of hydroxypropylcellulose decreased diffusivity of the drug in the matrix and increased matrix swelling. Polyvinylpirrolidone accelerated the release of pilocarpine by decreasing the matrix swelling by increasing surface attrition of the matrix (Urtti et al., 1985b).

Pilocarpine release and polymer dissolution were faster in matrices of ethyl than propyl and butyl half-esters of poly(vinyl methyl ether-maleic anhydride). The rates of pilocarpine release and polymer dissolution decreased with the decreased buffering capacity of the dissolution medium. Pilocarpine did not release from half-esters of poly(vinyl methyl ether-maleic anhydride) according to erosion-controlled mechanism: part of the drug diffuses from the uneroded portion of the matrices. Erosion-controlled drug release from the matrices of alkyl half-esters of poly(vinyl methyl ether-maleic anhydride) was not self-evident. It is obtained only as an ideal combination of properties of dissolution medium, drug and polymer (Urtti, 1985c).

In in vivo experiments with pigmented rabbits (Urtti, 1985d) the propyl half-ester of poly(vinyl methyl ether-maleic anhydride) matrices showed vehicle-controlled drug delivery. The matrices resulted in decreased magnitude and delayed onset of the peak miotic response (Table 1). In the tear fluid the ethyl half-ester dissolved in 3 h and the propyl half-ester in 8 h (Urtti, 1985d).

Table 1
Time delay (t_{max})and magnitude (RP_{max}) of the peak miotic response after administration of 0.6 mg of pilocarpine in 2.35% pilocarpine hydrochloride eye drops, and in matrices of ethyl and propyl half-esters of PVM-MA. Means ± S.E.M. of five determinations (Urtti, 1985d)

Dosage form	Vehicle	t_{max}(min)	RP_{max}
Eye drop	phosphate buffer (pH 6.4)	34.0 ± 6.9	2.066 ± 0.419
Matrix	ethyl half-ester of PVM-MA	87.0 ± 34.3	1.189 ± 0.345
Matrix	propyl half-ester of PVM-MA	142.0 ± 31.2*	0.638 ± 0.122*

* $P < 0.05$ compared to eye drops.
(Wilcoxon's matched pairs ranked signs test)

CLINICAL EXPERIENCES WITH PILOCARPINE INSERTS

Despite the fact that numerous erodible pilocarpine inserts have been presented in experimental studies only a few of them have been tested in human therapy.

Bensinger et al. (1976) administered pilocarpine (0.5, 1.0, 1.5 and 2.0 mg) to a selected group of ocular hypertensive subjects in the form of a synthetic biosoluble matrix inserted into the conjunctival cul-de-sac. Satisfactory lowering of the intraocular pressure resulted, with a minimum subject intolerance. Most of the side effects were those customarily associated with the administration of pilocarpine, such as tearing, blurring, fullness, soreness, and headache. The symptoms tended to increase as the inserted dose increased, although no patient reported the side effects to be as severe as their worst experience with pilocarpine drops. The decreased pressure response was significant in some cases for more than 24 hours. According to the authors drug delivery by soluble inserts offers promise as a convenient and effective mode of therapy.

In the USSR soluble ophthalmic drug inserts of ABE copolymer have been used for nearly a decade in human therapy for a broad spectrum of ocular drugs (Table 2)(Maichuk, 1976,1985). ABE copolymer is a macromolecule consisting of acrylamide, vinylpirrolidone and ethylacrylate residues (Maichuk, 1985).

Table 2
Soluble ophthalmic drug inserts in clinical or in preclinical use in the USSR (Maichuk, 1985)

Pilocarpine hydrochloride 2.7 mg
Pilocarpine hydrochloride 2.0 mg and adrenaline hydrotartrate 0.5 mg
Nivaline 2.0 mg
Timolol 0.5 mg and pilocarpine hydrochloride 2.5 mg
Florenal 0.2 mg
Idoxuridine 0.5 mg
Bromuridine 0.5 mg
Adenine-arabinoside 2.0 mg
Gludantan 0.2 mg
Dexamethasone 0.1 mg
Sodium sulfapyridazine 5.2 mg
Neomycin sulphate 1.12 mg
Kanamycin sulphate 1.2 mg
Gentamycin sulphate 1.5 mg
Kanamycin sulphate 1.5 mg and dexamethasone 0.005 mg
Taufon (taurine) 3.0 mg
Atropine sulphate 1.6 mg
Dicaine 0.75 mg
Sodium sulfapyridazine 0.9 mg and dicaine 0.5 mg
Fibrinolysin 400-450 AU

The Soviet inserts have recently been licensed by Diversified Technology Inc. (Salt Lake City, Utah) and are in the process of being registered in the western world (Lee and Robinson, 1986).

Pilocarpine inserts are oval-shaped thin homogeneous polymer platelets, colored green, 9x4.5x0.35 mm in size. The insert contains 2.7 mg pilocarpine hydrochloride. Placed in the inferior cul-de-sac the insert is quickly wetted by the lacrimal fluid to become plastic 10 to 15 s later and assumes the curved configuration of the eyeball. Within the following 10 to 15 min the film turns into a viscous polymer clot still retaining its shape. In the following 30 to 60 min it becomes a polymer solution. In pigmented rabbit and in human eyes the pilocarpine inserts induced maximal miosis within 10-20 min and it lasted longer than after aqueous and oily pilocarpine eye drops (Maichuk, 1985).

According to e.g. Maichuk and Erichev (1981) soluble ophthalmic drug insert with 2.7 mg of pilocarpine once daily effectively reduced intraocular pressure in 155 glaucoma patients. In only 8 of the 155 patients did pilocarpine inserts have to be discontinued because of individual intolerance causing lacrimation, pain in the eyes, and hyperemia of the conjunctiva.

EFFECT OF PILOCARPINE INSERTS ON PILOCARPINE PLASMA LEVELS

About 1% of the instilled dose of pilocarpine is absorbed into the eye (Chrai and Robinson, 1974). We studied (Urtti et al.,1985e) in the rabbit the systemic absorption of ocular pilocarpine after administration in aqueous solution, in hydroxypropylcellulose (HPC) matrix, and in a matrix of n-butyl half-ester of poly(vinyl methyl ether-maleic anhydride) (PVM-MA). In the inferior cul-de-sac, HPC matrices dissolved in 7-12 min. n-Butyl half-ester of PVM-MA neither dissolved totally nor released all the drug from the matrix in the tear fluid during 8 h. Besides improving ocular drug absorption, the pilocarpine concentration in systemic circulation was decreased from the 72% of the total dose observed after aqueous solution to 67% and 41% after HPC-matrix and matrix of n-butyl half-ester of PVM-MA, respectively. We suppose that systemic absorption of other ophthalmic drugs can be similarly modified with polymer matrices. Especially in children and in the elderly, the systemic absorption (e.g. Kaila et al., 1985) and side--effects of many ophthalmic drugs is a concern.

COMMENTS AND CHALLENGES

Despite considerable experimental work on pilocarpine soluble inserts the inserts are not - with the exception of those developed and used in the USSR - used in topical ocular drug delivery. None of the inserts showed vehicle-controlled pilocarpine delivery although those developed by Urtti (1985d) were more advanced. In the inferior cul-de-sac the inserts were generally gelled in minutes and dissolved in hours. The sustained miotic and intraocular pressure lowering effect of the pilocarpine inserts is partly due to rapid initial release of a large amount of pilocarpine saturating the corneal epithelium, which then becomes the drug reservoir rather than the insert. With present soluble inserts a prolonged pulse-entry of pilocarpine is obtained.

The study on the inserts has, however, greatly increased our understanding on drug disposition in the eye as well as given new challenges for topical ocular drug delivery. According to Lee and Robinson (1986) the efforts to improve ocular drug delivery ought to be concentrated on liquid systems, even though liquids are poorly retained in the eye. The inserts might, however, meet some of the new demands of ocular drug delivery: the noncorneal (conjunctival-scleral) absorption route (Ahmed and Patton, 1985) to target tissues in the anterior and posterior uvea and to the vitreous. In connection with intraocular operation with conjunctival flap soluble drug inserts delivering anti-inflammatory and microbial drugs might be placed under the conjunctiva instead of subconjunctival injections (with low ocular bioavailability). This route might also allow the delivery of macromolecules into the eye. From the point of view of pharmaceutical technology it might be possible to develop inserts to release drugs for weeks and even for months.

REFERENCES

Ahmed I, Patton TF (1985) Importance of the noncorneal absorption route in topical ophthalmic drug delivery. Invest Ophthalmol Vis Sci 26:584-587.

Bensinger R, Shin DH, Kass MA, Podos SM, Becker B (1976) Pilocarpine ocular inserts. Invest Ophthalmol 15:1008-1010.

Birss SA, Longwell A, Heckbert S, Keller N (1978) Ocular hypotensive efficacy of topical epinephrine in normotensive and hypertensive rabbits: continous drug delivery vs eyedrops. Ann Ophthalmol 10:1045-1054.

Bloomfield SE, Dunn MW, Miyata T, Stenzel KH (1977) Soluble gentamycin ophthalmic inserts as a drug delivery system. Arch Ophthalmol 95:247-250.

Chrai SS, Robinson JR (1974) Corneal penetration of topical pilocarpine nitrate in the rabbit. Am J Ophthalmol 77:735-739.

Dohlman CH, Pavan-Langston D, Rose J (1972) A new ocular insert for continuous constant-rate delivery of medication to the eye. Ann Ophthalmol 4:823-832.

Grass GM, Cobby J, Makoid MC (1984) Ocular delivery of pilocarpine from erodible matrices. J Pharm Sci 73:618-621.

Kaila T, Salminen L, Huupponen R (1985) Systemic absorption of topically applied ocular timolol. J Ocular Pharmacol 1:79-83.

Katz IM, Blackman WM (1977) A soluble sustained-release ophthalmic delivery unit. Amer J Ophthalmol 83:728-734.

Katz JI, Kaufman HE, Breslin C, Katz IM (1978) Slow-release artificial tears and the treatment of keratitis sicca. Ophthalmology 85:787-793.

Lee VHL, Robinson JR (1986) Review: Topical ocular drug delivery: recent developments and future challenges. J Ocular Pharmacol 2:67-108.

Lerman S (1970) Simulated sustained release pilocarpine therapy. Ann Ophthalmol 2:435-439.

Loucas SP, Haddad HM (1972) Solid-state ophthalmic dosage systems in effecting prolonged release of pilocarpine in the cul-de-sac. J Pharm Sci 61:985-986.

Maichuk YF (1976) Polymeric drug delivery systems in ophthalmology. In: Leopold IH, Burns RP (eds): Ocular therapy. John Wiley and Sons, New York; pp.1-16.

Maichuk YF, Erichev VP (1981) Soluble ophthalmic drug inserts with pilocarpine: experimental and clinical study. Glaucoma 3:239-242.

Maichuk YF (1985) Medicated eye films. Medexport, Moscow;pp.1-66.

Maurice DM, Mishima S (1984) Ocular pharmacokinetics. In: Sears ML (ed): Handbook of experimental pharmacology, Vol.69. Springer-Verlag, Berlin-Heidelberg; pp.19-116.

Mishima S (1981) Clinical pharmacokinetics of the eye. Invest Ophthalmol Vis Sci 21:504-541.

Pavan-Langston D, Langston RHS, Geary PA (1975) Idoxuridine ocular insert therapy. Arch Ophthalmol 93:1349-1351.

Richardson KT (1975) Ocular microtherapy. Membrane-controlled drug delivery. Arch Ophthalmol 93:74-86.

Saettone MF, Giannaccini B, Teneggi A, Savigni P, Tellini N (1982) Vehicle effects on ophthalmic bioavailability: the influence of different polymers on the activity of pilocarpine in rabbit and man. J Pharm Pharmacol 34:464-466.

Saettone MF, Giannaccini B, Chetoni P, Galli G, Chiellini E (1984) Vehicle effects in ophthalmic bioavailability: an evaluation of polymeric inserts containing pilocarpine. J Pharm Pharmacol 36:229-234.

Salminen L, Urtti A, Kujari H, Juslin M (1983) Prolonged pulse-entry of pilocarpine with a soluble drug inserts. Graefes Arch Clin Exp Ophthalmol 221:96-99.

Salminen L, Urtti A, Periviita L (1984) Effect of ocular pigmentation on pilocarpine pharmacology.I. Drug distribution and metabolism. Int J Pharm 18:17-24.

Shell JW (1984) Ophthalmic drug delivery systems. Surv Ophthalmol 29:117-128.

Urtti A, Salminen L, Kujari H, Jantti V (1984) Effect of ocular pigmentation on pilocarpine pharmacology in the rabbit eye.II. Drug response. Int J Pharm 19:53-61.

Urtti A, Periviita L, Salminen L, Juslin M (1985a) Effects of hydrophilicity of polymer matrix on in vitro release of pilocarpine and on its miotic activity in rabbit eyes. Drug Development and Industrial Pharmacy 11:257-268.

Urtti A, Juslin M, Miinalainen O (1985b) Pilocarpine release from hydroxypropylcellulose-polyvinylpirrolidone matrices. Int J Pharm 25:165-178.

Urtti A (1985c) Pilocarpine release from matrices of alkyl half-esters of poly(vinyl methyl ether-maleic anhydride). Int J Pharm 26:45-55.

Urtti A (1985d) Deliverial and pharmacokinetic aspects of ocular pilocarpine administration. University of Kuopio, Kuopio; pp.1-94.

Urtti A, Salminen L, Miinalainen O (1985e) Systemic absorption of ocular pilocarpine is modified by polymer matrices. Int J Pharm 23:147-161.

Yoshida S, Mishima S (1975) A pharmacokinetic analysis of the pupil response to topical pilocarpine and tropicamide. Jpn J Ophthalmol 19:121-138.

SURFACTANT PHARMACOKINETICS IN THE EYE

K. Green[1,2], L. Cheeks[1] and J.M. Chapman[1]

Department of Ophthalmology[1] and
Department of Physiology and Endocrinology[2],
Medical College of Georgia,
Augusta, Georgia 30912-0300 USA

The ocular pharmacokinetics of benzalkonium chloride (BAK) and sodium lauryl sulfate (SLS) have been determined in neonatal, young, and adult rabbits. BAK is confined to the cornea and conjunctiva, while SLS distributes widely. After single- or multiple-drop administration, the order of accumulation is neonatal > young > adult eye. Multiple-drop administration leads to accumulation to a tissue dependent steady state. BAK and SLS alter membrane permeability and can alter protein profiles of neonatal cells in culture. Such changes may alter tissue growth and differentiation.

Because of their bacteriocidal or bacteriostatic properties surfactants are widely used in commercial preparations in the ophthalmic, as well as the cosmetic, industry. In ophthalmology one of the primary surfactants used is the cationic agent, benzalkonium chloride. This material acts on bacteria by lysing cell walls, and because of this property it also enhances drug penetration through the cornea (O'Brien & Swan (1942); Green & Downs (1974); Green & Downs (1975)), both by actions on the epithelium (Green & Tonjum (1975); Tonjum (1977); Tonjum (1975)) and the endothelium (Green & Downs (1974); Green et al (1977)). These effects are seen with other cationic surfactants such as cetylpyridinium chloride (Green (1976); Godbey, Green & Hull (1979)). Non-ionic detergents have also been shown to enhance fluorescein penetration by up to as much as 5 times across the human cornea (Marsh & Maurice (1971)). Anionic surfactants, represented by sodium lauryl sulfate, are widely used in soaps and shampoos.

The pharmacokinetics of different classes of surfactants have only recently been examined in the eye (Clayton et al (1985); Green & Chapman (1986)), especially comparing neonatal, juvenile and adult eyes since only scant attention has been paid to pediatric dosing regimens (Green & Chapman (1986); Miller & Patton (1981)). This is of particular importance since actively growing and differentiating tissues in young eyes may be particularly susceptible to agents such as surfactants (Clayton et al (1985)) that may act as differentiation inducers and as teratogens. Knowledge of the pharmacokinetics of surfactants in the ocular tissues and fluids would enable the potential prediction of the impact of these agents on regularly treated eyes of the very young.

The methodology used in these experiments has been described in detail previously (Clayton et al (1985); Green & Chapman (1986)). The animals used were either albino or pigmented rabbits that were either neonates, juveniles or adults. Neonatal animals ranged from 3 to 4 weeks old and weighed less than 500 grams: these animals were born in our facility and studies were initiated within 5 or 6 days after their eyes had opened. Juvenile animals varied in weight from 500 to 1000 grams and were about 6 weeks old, while adult animals weighed between 2 and 3 kg.

The surfactants used were ^{14}C-benzalkonium chloride (specific activity 4.3

Ophthalmic Drug Delivery. Biopharmaceutical, Technological and Clinical Aspects.
M.S. Saettone, G. Bucci, P. Speiser (eds.) Fidia Research Series, vol. 11, Liviana Press, Padova © 1987

μCi/mg) and ^{35}S-sodium lauryl sulfate (specific activity 7.9 Ci/mmole), both synthesized by New England Nuclear Corporation, Boston, MA. Benzalkonium chloride was a C-23 compound with a C-14 alkyl chain. Benzalkonium chloride was applied topically as a 0.03% solution (0.02% radioactive material added to a 0.01% non-radioactive benzalkonium chloride containing solution, Tearisol, CooperVision) in juvenile and adult rabbits or at 0.02% (0.01% ^{14}C-benzalkonium chloride) in neonatal rabbits. Sodium lauryl sulfate was used at a 1.3% final concentration in a proprietary detergent formulation that contained no cationic detergents. All neonatal animals received drops of 10 μl; sodium lauryl sulfate was also applied as 10 μl drops; benzalkonium chloride was applied to the eyes of juvenile or adult rabbits in 50 μl drops. Various regimens of drop application were used, ranging from single drops to up to 22 drops given at 3 drops per day (for a total of 7 days of treatment). During multiple drop treatment, the last drop was given 1 hour prior to tissue and fluid sampling for direct comparison with data obtained 1 hour after single drop administration.

The tissue isolation procedures have also been described previously (Clayton et al (1985); Green & Chapman (1986)). Briefly, both eyes were taken for tissue and fluid sampling even though only one eye was treated. The ocular surface was washed with at least 1 ml of 0.9% saline before tissue or fluid samples were taken. In order of removal, the tissues and fluids harvested for analysis were: aqueous humor (taken by paracentesis), corneal epithelium (scraped from the cornea with a Gill corneal knife), palpebral and bulbar conjunctiva, the rest of the cornea (stroma plus endothelium), lens, iris-ciliary body, vitreous, choroid and retina. A plasma sample was obtained by direct cardiac puncture, and systemic tissues were also collected. All tissues and fluids were weighed, digested in Protosol, hydrogen peroxide added (to decolor the samples, except for aqueous humor; additionally, the pH of the lens samples was reduced by adding 1 N HCl), and Aquasol added before cooling of the samples for at least 24 hours before counting. Appropriate background counts and quench curves were used in data compilation.

Benzalkonium chloride (BAK).

No difference was found between albino and pigmented rabbits for the ocular distribution of BAK. This is caused by the limited ocular penetration of BAK since it is confined to non-pigmented tissues, namely the corneal epithelium, the stroma/endothelium and the palpebral and bulbar conjunctiva (Table 1). The values for tissues and fluids shown in Table 1 represent only those in which BAK was found after topical administration. At times when peak concentrations are found after a single drop, or even after multiple drop applications in both juveniles and adult rabbits BAK is confined first only to the treated eye, and second only to those tissues (cornea and conjunctiva) of the ocular surface (Table 1). Only in neonates after multiple drop application is any trace of BAK found in the aqueous humor, or the contralateral untreated eye (Table 2).

The time course of loss of BAK from those tissues into which BAK does penetrate is such that about a half of the 30 minute BAK concentration remained at 24 hours, and measurable values exist for up to 120 hours after a single drop administration. Tissues with the highest concentrations were the corneal epithelium and the palpebral conjunctiva (Table 1). In addition, major differences exist between juvenile and adult rabbits in terms of the peak concentrations of BAK with juvenile rabbits reaching much higher levels. Also, the rate of loss of BAK was faster from juvenile, compared to adult tissues, because the values at later times (72 and 120 hours) were quite smaller despite the considerably higher values at early times after drop instillation.

Multiple drop administration to juvenile rabbits leads to the rapid accumulation of BAK that reaches an equilibrium at different times in different tissues. The corneal epithelium, for instance, reaches an apparent equilibrium after 10 drops (72 hours, 3 drops a day, last drop 1 hour before tissue sampling) while the conjunctival (palpebral and bulbar) tissues reach an equilibrium after only 4 drops (3 drops one day, 4th drop on next day at 24 hours after first drop). Adult rabbits treated similarly also show accumulation of BAK although quantitatively the amounts were less (Green and Chapman (1986)). Neonatal animals, despite receiving drops that were only one-fifth the size, and two-thirds the BAK concentration, of those given to adult or juvenile rabbits also showed substantial accumulation of BAK, with tissue values being comparable to those found in juvenile rabbits. This indicated that neonatal animals have great avidity for these surfactants. Only with neonatal animals were even traces of BAK found in the contralateral eye.

Table 1.
Benzalkonium chloride distribution in the eye after single drop.

Time(hr)	Corneal Epithelium	Rest of Cornea	Palpebral Conjunctiva	Bulbar Conjunctiva
Juveniles:				
0.25	51 ± 9	1.0 ± 0.1	53 ± 11	23 ± 4
0.5	44 ± 11	0.7 ± 0.1	58 ± 6	14 ± 3
1	37 ± 6	0.8 ± 0.2	47 ± 4	18 ± 3
2	36 ± 5	0.7 ± 0.2	47 ± 4	11 ± 2
8	32 ± 7	1.0 ± 0.2	41 ± 3	15 ± 3
24	23 ± 3	1.1 ± 0.3	36 ± 3	11 ± 2
72	8 ± 2	0.4 ± 0.1	12 ± 1	7 ± 1
120	2 ± 0.8	0.4 ± 0.1	6.6 ± 0.7	3.1 ± 0.8
Adults:				
0.25	49 ± 12	0.6 ± 0.2	34 ± 5	4 ± 1
0.5	21 ± 2	0.4 ± 0.2	33 ± 7	14 ± 3
1	21 ± 8	0.5 ± 0.1	23 ± 6	9 ± 2
2	20 ± 5	0.5 ± 0.2	13 ± 3	5 ± 1
8	9 ± 1	0.3 ± 0.04	18 ± 4	8 ± 2
24	8 ± 2	0.3 ± 0.1	16 ± 3	11 ± 1
72	3 ± 0.5	0.1 ± 0.04	8 ± 1	5 ± 0.5
120	2 ± 1	0.1 ± 0.03	6 ± 1	4 ± 1

All values are the mean ± SEM (ng/mg tissue or fluid) for 5 tissues. Adapted from Green and Chapman (1986). Time is that elapsed since application of drops.

Sodium lauryl sulfate (SLS).

Unlike BAK, sodium lauryl sulfate (SLS) is widely distributed in ocular and systemic tissues and fluids even after a single drop administration (Clayton et al (1985)). SLS readily entered the eye and reached all ocular tissues and plasma within 30 minutes of drop application. In all cases, corneas showed the highest concentration, with choroid, retina and iris having sequentially lesser amounts. Penetration, presumably through the plasma, occurred into the untreated contralateral eye (Table 3). As with BAK, differences existed in both the rate and extent of uptake into tissues. The younger the animal, then the greater the amount of uptake. Even 48 hours after single drop administration substantial amounts of SLS remained in the ocular tissues, indicating a very slow washout. Tissue distribution of SLS was also different between different age groups, since, although the choroid, cornea and vitreous, of juvenile and neonatal animals contained similar quantities after multiple drop application (see Table 3), the retinal, lens and aqueous humor concentrations were much greater (at least twice) for neonatal rabbits.

Table 2.
Benzalkonium chloride distribution in the eye after single or multiple drop administration.

	Neonates	Juveniles[+]			
	16 drops	1 drop	4 drops	10 drops	16 drops
Aqueous humor	0.007 ±0.002	0	0	0	0
Corneal Epithelium	155 ± 23	37 ± 6	63 ± 4	200 ±36	186 ±23
Rest of Cornea	6.0 ±0.4	0.8 ±0.2	2.6 ±0.4	6.0 ±0.7	8.0 ±1.3
Palpebral Conjunctiva	58 ± 7	47 ± 4	81 ± 6	85 ± 6	61 ± 4
Bulbar Conjunctiva	24 ± 2	68 ± 3	50 ± 8	68 ± 8	58 ± 7
Plasma	80 ± 20	0	0	0	0

All values are the mean ± SEM (ng/mg tissue or fluid) of at least 5 eyes after each drop application regimen. + Data adapted from Green and Chapman (1986). Juveniles and adults received 50 µl drops of 0.03% BAK, neonates received 10 µl drops containing 0.02% BAK.

Multiple drop administration of SLS (Table 3) led to the accumulation of substantial amounts of the detergent with most tissues (cornea, epithelium, lens, and all systemic tissues) reaching an apparent equilibrium after 13 drops (4 days) administration, but some tissues (e.g., iris) showing continued accumulation even after 22 drops (7 days). The widespread systemic distribution of SLS is illustrated in Table 3, where accumulation also occurs to apparent equilibrium after 13 drops (4 days) of application. SLS is also found in varying amounts in the contralateral eye, at either low (iris, vitreous) or high concentrations (conjunctiva, cornea) but in no case does the contralateral eye concentration (even after multiple drop application) approach the value in the treated eye. From the data in Table 3, it is readily apparent that the contralateral eye can contain as much as 25% (in the case of the lens), or as little as 3% (in the case of the cornea) of the treated eye amount. It seems apparent that the high plasma levels can account for the distribution to the contralateral eye.

There is a great disparity in the ocular and systemic distribution of BAK and SLS. The cationic surfactant, BAK, is confined solely to the anterior ocular surface tissues, namely the corneal epithelium, rest of cornea and conjunctiva in all ages of animals except neonates where small, trace amounts are found in the aqueous humor and plasma with equally small amounts in the contralateral, untreated eye. This latter finding was true only after the application of multiple drops to the neonates. On the other hand, the anionic surfactant, SLS, is widely distributed in all ocular and all systemic tissues (at least of those that were sampled) even after single drop administration.

Table 3.
Sodium lauryl sulfate concentrations in ocular and systemic tissues and fluids after topical administration to the eye of albino rabbits.

		Neonates			Juveniles*
		1 drop	13 drops	22 drops	13 drops (72 hrs)
A	T	159± 14	364± 34	317± 34	172 ± 27
	C	27± 9	117± 8	65± 10	11 ± 0.4
CE	T	571704±101330	180572± 27280	157859± 20398	-
	C	2135± 993	892± 731	402± 142	-
RC	T	12368± 1466	15636± 2309	19853± 2997	19500 ±4000
	C	2074± 825	653± 65	659± 171	268 ± 86
L	T	144± 46	278± 31	176± 17(4)	135 ± 17
	C	79± 12(4)	138± 36	47± 2(4)	5.8± 0.6
I	T	488± 285	645± 316	1507± 452	1789 ± 729
	C	0(3)	0(4)	281± 29(4)	37 ± 4.4
V	T	26± 4(4)	86± 15	56± 11	63 ± 20
	C	11± 3(4)	49± 7	34± 4	2.4± 0.2
R	T	748± 138	735± 153	85± 176	5129 ±2444
	C	25± 10	56± 17	79± 20	20 ± 1
Ch	T	1917± 457	4057± 1531	3100± 658	3850 ±1194
	C	44± 22	143± 84	603± 238	73 ± 34
BC	T	36399± 5568	41619± 14133	22529± 3376	-
	C	1546± 359	884± 113	1137± 394	-
PC	T	12110± 2124	17726± 2149	14095± 1816	-
	C	243± 71	530± 53	404± 35	-
Kidney		894± 304	1515± 306	738± 107	187 ± 24
Liver		885± 280	1129± 217	701± 124	120 ± 9
Brain		21± 9(4)	40± 14	32± 10	39 ± 11
Heart		63± 32(4)	70± 17	67± 18	22 ± 6
Spleen		0(3)	111± 36	104± 13	21 ± 2
Plasma		130± 54	288± 18	220± 28	20 ± 0.1

All values are the mean ± SEM (pg/mg tissue or fluid) of at least 5 eyes 1 hour after the application of 1 drop, 13 drops, or 22 drops at 3 drops per day, last drop 1 hour before tissue harvesting on last day. * Data adapted from Clayton et al. (1985). A, aqueous humor; CE, corneal epithelium; RC, rest of cornea; L, lens; I, iris-ciliary processes; V, vitreous; R, retina; Ch, choroid; BC, bulbar conjunctiva; PC, palpebral conjunctiva.

Single drop administration of both BAK and SLS leads to rapid accumulation in the corneal epithelium and conjunctiva from where the surfactants are lost to either the tear film, probably exclusively in the case of BAK, or to the tears and to other tissues in the case of SLS. BAK must leach out of the epithelium and conjunctiva at a rate slow enough that it cannot be detected in the plasma. The only exception to this is in the neonatal animals receiving multiple drop administration where, after a total of 16 drops given over the course of 5 complete days, very small amounts were found both in the plasma and in the contralateral eye. The time course of loss for both BAK and SLS from the eye after a single drop is such that even after 48 or 72 hours considerable amounts remain in the tissues into which they penetrate. This behavior differs from many ophthalmic drugs that are often lost rapidly from the eye after topical administration (Green & Downs (1974); Green & Downs (1975); Miller & Patton (1981); Wei, Anderson & Leopold (1978); Araie et al (1982)). These surfactants, therefore, show quite different pharmacokinetic behavior compared to many other topically applied agents.

Multiple drop administration leads to accumulation of both surfactants in ocular (and, in the case of SLS, systemic) tissues, although for BAK the penetration is limited to the surface tissues. In neonatal animals, however, trace amounts of BAK can be found in the contralateral eye and in the plasma, indicating that in the very young rabbit sufficient BAK can be administered to reach a point where some systemic absorption occurs. Several tissues appear to reach an equilibrium with the applied doses of surfactants at the dosing regimen used here. The equilibrium tends to be reached earlier in tissues of younger animals, and varies from tissue to tissue.

The data obtained in these studies indicate that more surfactant is accumulated, from either single or multiple drop application, in tissues of younger compared to those of older animals. Such enhanced tissue uptake may reflect an increased permeability of either the cellular, or epithelial, membranes of younger animals, as well as the different properties of cells that make up the rapidly growing and differentiating tissues. The enhanced uptake of both BAK and SLS in tissues of very young animals may allow the tissue concentrations to reach a point where they can influence the properties of the cells. In primary cell culture, for example, we have found that cells from juvenile ocular tissues occasionally show restricted modification of the protein profile in the presence of either anionic or cationic surfactants (Clayton et al (1985)).

The results suggest that the use of surfactants that come into contact with the eye, either by choice, as in the case of BAK included as a bacteriocide in topical ophthalmic medications, or by accident, as in the use of SLS in soaps and shampoos, should by minimized. These compounds are known to alter cell and epithelial membrane permeability (Green & Downs (1974); Green & Downs (1975); Green & Tonjum (1975); Tonjum (1977); Tonjum (1975); Green et al (1977); Green (1976); Godbey, Green & Hull (1979); Marsh & Maurice (1971)) and also alter protein profiles (Clayton et al (1985)) and such changes might alter the growth and differentiation of these tissues.

ACKNOWLEDGEMENTS.

Supported in part by research grant from the National Eye Institute (EY04558), in part by a Senior International Fellowship (F06TW00687) from the Fogarty International Center of the National Institutes of Health (both to KG), in part by the American Medical Association, Education and Research Foundation (JMC), and in part by a departmental award from Research to Prevent Blindness, Inc. We thank Sylvia Catravas and Lynne Nichols for their invaluable secretarial assistance.

REFERENCES

Araie M, Tabase M, Sakai Y, Ishii Y, Yokoyama Y, and Kitagawa M (1982) Beta adrenergic blockers: Ocular penetration and binding to uveal pigment. Jap J Ophthalmol. 26: 248-263.

Clayton RM, Green K, Wilson M, Zehir A, Jack J and Searle L (1985) The penetration of detergents into adult and infant eyes: Possible hazards of additives to ophthalmic preparations. Fd Chem Tox 23: 239-246.

Godbey REW, Green K and Hull DS (1979) Influence of cetylpyridinium chloride on corneal permeability to penicillin. J Pharm Sci 68: 1176-1180.

Green K (1976) Electrophysiological and anatomical effects of cetylpyridinium chloride on the rabbit cornea. Acta Ophthalmol (Kbh) 54: 145-159.

Green K and Chapman JM (1986) Benzalkonium chloride kinetics in young and adult albino and pigmented rabbit eyes. J Toxicol Cutan Ocular Toxicol 5: 132-142.

Green K and Downs S (1974) Prednisolone phosphate penetration into and through the cornea. Invest Ophthalmol 13: 316-319.

Green K and Downs S (1975) Ocular penetration of pilocarpine in rabbits. Arch Ophthalmol 93: 1165-1168.

Green K, Hull DS, Vaughn E, Malizia A and Bowman K (1977) Rabbit endothelial response to ophthalmic preservatives. Arch Ophthalmol 95: 2218-2221.

Green K and Tonjum AM (1975) The effect of benzalkonium chloride on the electropotential of the rabbit cornea. Acta Ophthalmol (Kbh) 53: 348-357.

Marsh RJ and Maurice DM (1971) Influence of non-ionic detergents and other surfactants on human corneal permeability. Exp Eye Res 11: 43-48.

Miller SC and Patton TF (1981) Age-related differences in ophthalmic drug disposition: I. Effect of size on the intraocular tissue distribution in albino rabbits. Biopharm Drug Dispos 2: 215-233.

O'Brien CS and Swan KC (1942) Carbaminoylcholine chloride in the treatment of glaucoma simplex. Arch Ophthalmol 27: 253-263.

Patton TF (1977) Pediatric dosing considerations in ophthalmology: dosage adjustments based on aqueous humor volume ratio. J Ped Ophthalmol 14: 254-256.

Tonjum AM (1975) Effects of benzalkonium chloride upon the corneal epithelium studied with scanning electron microscopy. Acta Ophthalmol (Kbh) 53: 358-366.

Tonjum AM (1977) Permeability of the rabbit corneal epithelium to horseradish peroxidase after the influence of benzalkonium chloride. Acta Ophthalmol (Kbh) 54: 335-347.

Wei C, Anderson JA and Leopold I (1978) Ocular absorption and metabolism of topically applied epinephrine and a dipivalyl ester of epinephrine. Invest Ophthalmol Vis Sci 17: 315-321.

CONTROLLED DRUG RELEASE FROM MONOLITHIC SYSTEMS

J. Heller

Polymer Sciences Department
SRI International, Menlo Park, CA 94025, USA

Controlled drug release from monolithic systems can be achieved by diffusion, swelling, or erosion. In diffusion-controlled systems the drug is dissolved or dispersed in a polymer matrix and allowed to diffuse from the monolith. In swelling-controlled systems the drug is immobilized in a glassy, hydrophilic polymer and is released as a swelling front moves into the matrix. In chemically controlled systems, rate of drug release is controlled by a combination of diffusion and erosion or in special cases, by erosion alone.

This brief review will be limited to drug delivery devices in which the therapeutic agent is physically dispersed in a polymer matrix and where the rate-controlling mechanism is diffusion, polymer swelling, or polymer erosion. The review will not cover devices where the therapeutic agent is chemically attached to a polymer or where the therapeutic agent is contained in a reservoir surrounded by a rate-controlling membrane. Further, it will not cover osmotically driven devices.

DIFFUSION CONTROLLED DEVICES

In a diffusion controlled monolithic device the therapeutic agent is intimately mixed in a rate-controlling polymer, and release occurs by diffusion of the agent from the polymer. It is necessary to consider two types of devices. In one, the active agent is dissolved in the polymer, whereas in the other, the active agent is dispersed in the polymer.

For an active agent dissolved in the matrix, release kinetics can be calculated by two equations (Baker and Lonsdale, 1974). Equation (1), known as the early time approximation, holds true for the first 60% of the release rate, after which it is calculated from equation (2), which is known as the late time approximation.

$$\frac{dM_t}{dt} = 2M_\infty \left(\frac{D}{\pi \ell^2 t} \right)^{1/2} \tag{1}$$

$$\frac{dM_t}{dt} = \frac{8DM_\infty}{\ell^2} \exp \left(- \frac{\pi^2 Dt}{\ell^2} \right) \tag{2}$$

Ophthalmic Drug Delivery. Biopharmaceutical, Technological and Clinical Aspects.
M.S. Saettone, G. Bucci, P. Speiser (eds.) Fidia Research Series, vol. 11, Liviana Press, Padova © 1987

These equations predict active agent release rate from a slab of thickness ℓ where D is the diffusion coefficient, M_∞ is the total amount of active agent dissolved in the polymer and M_t is the amount released at time t. As equation (1) shows, release rate decreases as $t^{-1/2}$ over the first 60% of the release; over the remainder of the release the rate decays exponentially according to equation (2). Plots of these two approximations are shown in Figure 1.

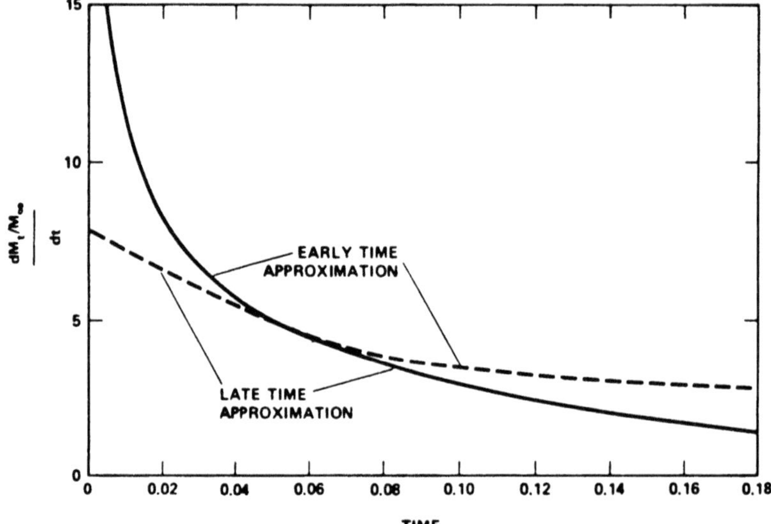

Figure 1. Plots of the release rate of drug initially dissolved in a slab as a function of time, using the early time and late time approximations. Reproduced with permission from Baker RW, Lonsdale HK (1974); Tanquery AC, Lacy RF (eds.); Controlled release of biologically active agents. Plenum Press, New York; pp 15-71.

For active agents dispersed in the polymer, release kinetics can be calculated from the Higuchi equation (Higuchi, 1961).

$$\frac{dM_t}{dt} = \frac{A}{2}\left[\frac{2DC_sC_o}{t}\right]^{1/2} \qquad (3)$$

where A is the area, C_s is the solubility of the active agent in the matrix and C_o is total concentration in the matrix (dissolved plus dispersed).

Unlike the slab with dissolved active agent in which the rate is proportional to $t^{-1/2}$ only during the early portion of the release curve, slabs with dispersed active agent maintain a $t^{-1/2}$ dependence over the major portion of the release curve and deviate from this dependence only when the concentration of the active agent remaining in the matrix falls below the saturation value. In these systems, a plot of cumulative release versus $t^{-1/2}$ yields a straight line.

The nonlinear release kinetics typical of diffusional monolithic systems are due to the formation of an increasing thickness of drug depleted polymer through which remaining drug must diffuse and this process is shown in Figure 2 for the diffusion of a steroid from a poly(dimethyl siloxane) matrix.

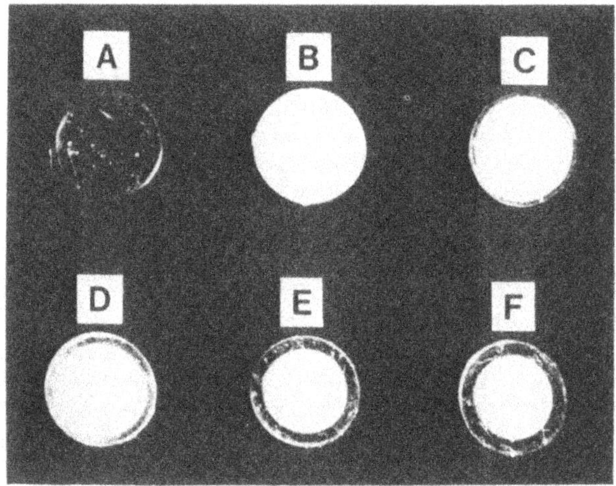

Figure 2. Cross-sectional views of silicone (transparent) cylinders. Key: A = placebo; B = drug-filled initial; C = 1 week; D = 2 weeks; E = 3 weeks; F = 4 weeks. Reproduced with permission from Roseman TJ, Higuchi WI (1970). Release of medroxyprogesterone acetate from a silicone polymer. J. Pharm. Sci. 59: 353-357

Monolithic diffusional devices can be modified to achieve release kinetics approximating zero order. In one such modification a hemisphere is constructed and coated on all sides except a circular opening in the center face with an impermeable coating (Hsieh, Rhine, and Langer, 1983). In these devices the effect of increasing thickness of drug depleted polymer is offset by the increasing surface area of drug containing polymer. Release kinetics from such a device compared to that of an ordinary slab are shown in Figure 3.

In another modification a device is constructed in which drug concentration in the matrix increases from the outer layers inwards and this increasing drug concentration offsets the effect of increasing thickness of drug depleted polymer layers (Lee, 1985). The non-uniform drug concentration is achieved by using a solvent leaching technique. Drug release from such devices as a function of the non-uniform drug distribution is shown in Figure 4. Therapeutically important devices are constructed using hydrophilic polymers and a water leaching technique.

SWELLING CONTROLLED DEVICES

In swelling-controlled systems an active agent is homogeneously dispersed in a glassy polymer. Because glassy polymers are essentially drug impermeable, the active agent is immobilized in the matrix, and no diffusion through the solid polymer takes place.

When such a monolithic device is placed in an aqueous environment, water begins to penetrate the matrix and swelling takes place. As a consequence of the swelling process, chain relaxation takes place, and the incorporated active agent begins to diffuse from the swollen layer.

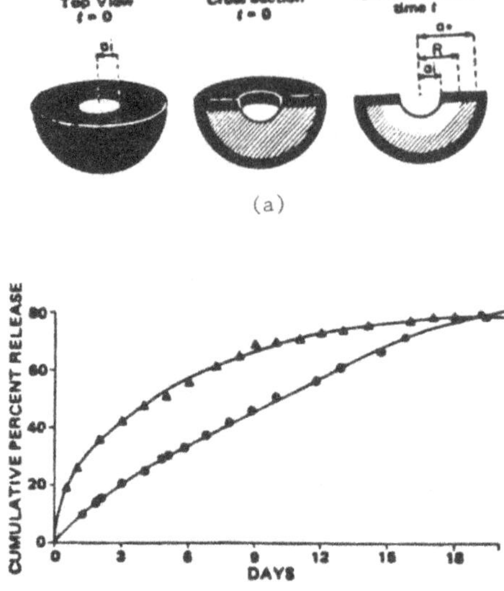

Figure 3. (a) Diagram of an inwardly-releasing hemisphere; a_i is the inner radius, a_o is the outer radius, and R is the distance to the interface between the dissolved region (white area) and the dispersed zone (diagonal lines). Black represents laminated regions through which release cannot occur.

(b) Cumulative release of sodium salicylate versus time for the geometric shapes made as described in the text. Key: (●) hemisphere, (▲) slabs. Reproduced with permission from Hsieh DST, Rhine WP, Langer R (1983). Zero order controlled release polymer matrices for micro and macromolecules, J. Pharm. Sci. 72: 17-22

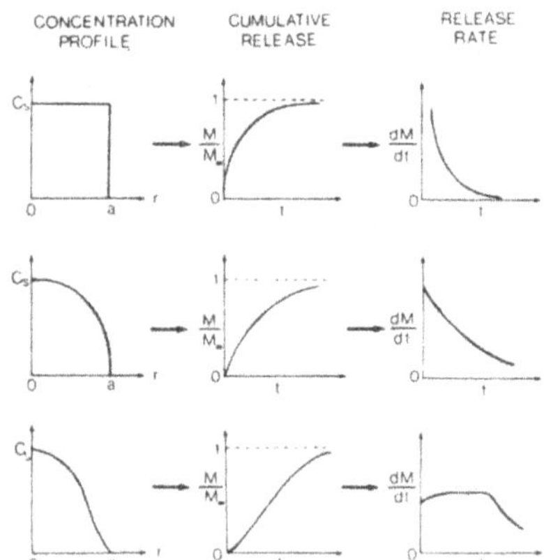

Figure 4. Theoretical profiles illustrating the effect of inital drug concentration distribution on the characteristics of drug release. Reprinted with permission from Lee PI (1985). Kinetics of drug release from hydrogel matrices. J. Controlled Release 2: 277-288

This process is represented schematically in Figure 5 (Langer and Peppas, 1983). One front separating the glassy from the rubbery state moves inward while a second front separating the swollen rubbery polymer from the surrounding aqueous environment moves outward.

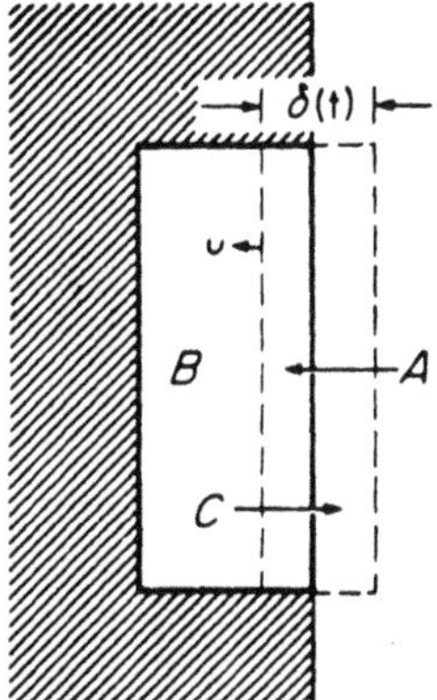

Figure 5. Schematic representation of swelling-controlled release system. As the penetrant A enters the glassy polymer B, bioactive agent C is released through the gel phase of thickness δ(t). Reprinted with permission from Langer R, Peppas N (1983). Chemical and physical structure of polymers as carriers for controlled release of biologically active agents: a review. Rev. Macromol. Chem. Phys. C23: 61-126.

In linear amorphous polymers, dissolution follows the swelling process, but crosslinked polymers or those containing significant chain entanglements or partial crystallinity will remain insoluble but will be mechanically weak.

CHEMICALLY CONTROLLED DEVICES

In a chemically controlled monolithic device, rate of active agent release is controlled by a chemical reaction that leads to polymer solubilization or degradation to small, water-soluble products. In such systems, kinetics of drug release depends on whether the polymer undergoes bulk hydrolysis or whether the hydrolysis is confined to the outer surface of the device (Heller, 1980). Because kinetics of release are different for these two systems, they will be discussed separately.

Bulk Hydrolysis - in this process hydrolysis occurs throughout the bulk of the polymer, and in general, an analysis of kinetics of drug release is complex because it combines diffusion and polymer hydrolysis. Thus, because bulk hydrolysis changes the matrix, permeability of the polymer to the drug will increase with time, but this increase is not predictable, and the increase in drug release rate is also not predictable. Furthermore, the matrix can disintegrate before drug depletion has taken place and a large burst in drug delivery can occur.

The most extensively investigated hydrophobic bulk eroding polymers are poly(lactic acid) and copolymers of glycolic and lactic acids (Heller, 1984). These polymers were originally developed as bioerodible sutures (Kulkarni, Pani, Neuman, and Leonard, 1966; Frazza and Schmitt, 1971); and degrade to the natural metabolites glycolic or lactic acid. Thus, they satisfy the requirement of degrading to toxicologically innocuous products and for this reason they occupy a preeminent place among bioerodible polymers.

Studies of the release of norethindrone from poly(lactic acid) and copolymers of lactic and glycolic acid illustrate the effect of bulk hydrolysis on release rate of an incorporated drug. Thus, Figure 6 shows release of norethindrone measured as serum level in baboons from poly(lactic acid) microspheres (Beck et al., 1981). Because drug depletion takes place before any significant polymer hydrolysis has taken place, kinetics of drug release are identical to those from a nonerodible monolithic system as already described.

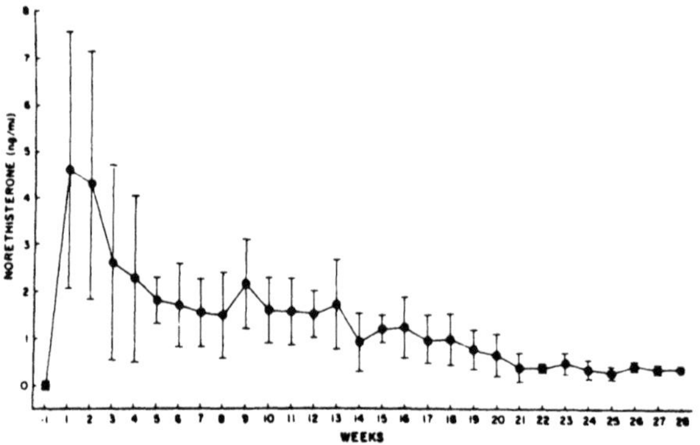

Figure 6. Peripheral mean serum levels of immune-reactive NET in seven human subjects following intramuscular injection of microcapsules containing 25% NET. The mean dose of NET = 87.21 ± 9.12 mg or 1.5 ± 0.37 mg of NET per kilogram of body weight. Reprinted with permission from Beck LR et al (1981). Clinical evaluation of injectable biodegradable contraceptive system. Am. J. Obstet. Gynecol. 140: 799-806.

However, if the more rapidly eroding copolymer of lactic and glycolic acid is used, release kinetics shown in Figure 7 are obtained (Beck et al., 1983). Here, during the early stages where little polymer hydrolysis has taken place, rate of drug release follows $t^{-1/2}$ kinetics and is determined by simple diffusion. However, as the polymer begins to hydrolyze, release rate accelerates because it is now controlled by a combination of diffusion and polymer hydrolysis.

Surface Hydrolysis - In surface hydrolysis, the process is confined to the outer surface of the device while the interior remains essentially unchanged.

Unlike bulk hydrolysis, where release rates of incorporated drugs are neither constant nor predictable, in systems undergoing surface hydrolysis, drug release is constant provided diffusional release is minimal and the device maintains a constant surface geometry. Furthermore, because release of the drug occurs as a direct consequence of the hydrolysis process, release rates are predictable if hydrolysis of the polymer is understood. Additional advantages of surface erosion is that rate of drug release is directly proportional to drug loading, and because erosion occurs by the movement of an eroding front, lifetime of the device is directly proportional to device thickness. Also, because release from the device does not involve diffusion, surface eroding systems are capable of releasing macromolecules at constant and predictable rates.

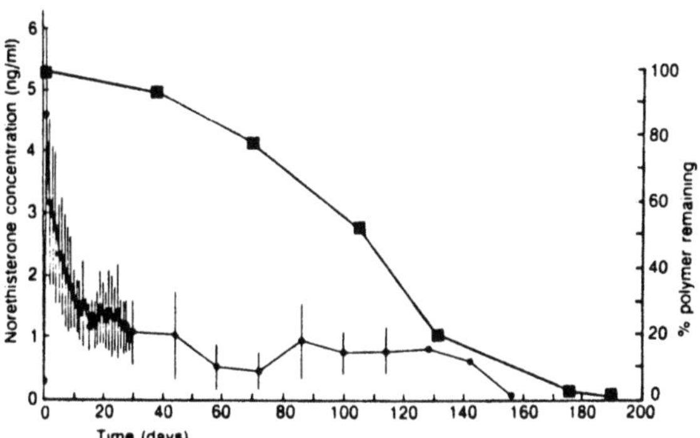

Figure 7. Mean ± SD serum levels of immunoreactive norethindrone (norethisterone) in five women treated by intramuscular injection of sterilized microcapsules (mean dose = 1.027 ± 0.1228 mg of norethindrone per kilogram). Top line represents biodegradation of the polymer. Reprinted with permission from Beck LR et al. (1983). Clinical evaluation of an improved injectable microcapsule contraceptive system. Am. J. Obstet. Gynecol. 147: 815-821

At present, there are three polymer systems with demonstrated surface erosion characteristics. These are partially esterified copolymers of methyl vinyl ether and maleic anhydride, poly(ortho esters), and polyanhydrides.

Partially esterified copolymers of methyl vinyl ether and maleic anhydride were the first reported example of surface-eroding polymers and solubilize by an ionization of carboxylic acid groups (Heller, Baker, Gale, and Rodin, 1978).

$$\underset{\text{insoluble}}{\left[-CH_2-\underset{}{CH}(OCH_3)-CH(C(=O)OR)-CH(C(=O)OH)-\right]_n} \longrightarrow \underset{\text{soluble}}{\left[-CH_2-CH(OCH_3)-CH(C(=O)OR)-CH(C(=O)O^-)-\right]_n \; H^+}$$

Because these polymers undergo a dissolution process without backbone cleavage they are only useful in topical applications where elimination of a high molecular weight, water-soluble polymer can proceed with no difficulty. One such application are bioerodible ocular inserts where a flat polymer disc containing dispersed therapeutic agent is placed in the lower cul-de-sac of the eye where it undergoes a dissolution process with concomitant drug release.

The usefulness of this approach has been demonstrated by placing hydrocortisone-containing devices in the lower forniceal cul-de-sac of New Zealand rabbits, removing devices at periodic intervals and determining residual drug remaining in the devices. Results of that study are shown in Figure 8. Clearly, the device is highly functional and even though every data point represents a separate device and a separate rabbit, there is remarkably little a scatter.

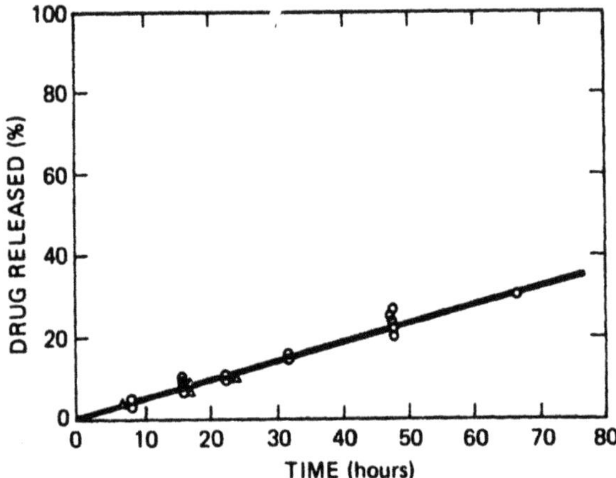

Figure 8. Release of hydrocortisone from ocular inserts in rabbits. Reprinted with permission from Heller J, Baker RW (1980); Baker RW (ed.). Controlled release of bioactive materials, Academic Press, New York, pp 1-17

The second surface-eroding polymer system are poly(ortho esters). These are prepared by adding alcohols to diketene acetals (Heller, Penhale, and Helwing, 1980) shown schematically as follows:

```
     OR          OR                                  OR          OR
     |           |                                   |           |
CH2=C-O-R'-O-C=CH2  +  HO-R"-OH  ---->  [ -O-C-O-R'-O-C-O-R"- ]n
                                             |           |
                                             CH3         CH3
```

Even though this is a condensation polymerization, no small molecules by-products are evolved so that dense, crosslinked matrices can be produced by using varying proportions of monomers having a functionality greater than two.

Principally because of ease of monomer synthesis, polymers were prepared by adding various diols to 3,9-bis(methylene 2,4,8,10-tetraoxaspiro [5,5] undecane) where R = H or to 3,9-bis(ethylidene-2,4,8,10-tetraoxaspiro [5,5] undecane) where R = CH_3:

```
        O-CH2      CH2-O                         [ RCH    O-CH2     CH2      CHR  ]
       /     \    /     \                        [   \   /     \   /   \    /     ]
RCH=C         C          C=CHR  +  HO-R-OH       [    C         C        C        ]
       \     /    \     /                        [   /   \     /   \    /  \      ]
        O-CH2      CH2-O                         [ -O     O-CH2     CH2-O    O-R- ]n
```

The ultimate degradation products are diol, pentaerithrytol and either acetic or propionic acids.

Because the polymer is acid sensitive, rate of polymer erosion can be manipulated within a very wide range by means of excipients physically incorporated into the matrix (Heller, Penhale, Fritzinger, and Ng, 1984). Thus, delivery devices having lifetimes between hours and a few weeks can be prepared by using acidic excipients such as anhydrides (Sparer, Shih, Ringeisen, and Himmelstein, 1984) or by using 9,10-dihydroxystearic acid as one of the monomers which yields polymers having pendant carboxylic acid groups (Heller, Penhale, Fritzinger, and Ng, 1987).

Delivery devices having lifetimes of months to years can be prepared by stabilizing the interior of the matrix with a base such as $Mg(OH)_2$ so that only the surface layers can erode where the $Mg(OH)_2$ has been neutralized by the external medium (Heller, Fritzinger, Ng, and Penhale, 1985). Figure 9 shows levonorgestrel blood plasma levels in rabbits with implanted devices using the basic excipient $Mg(OH)_2$ in a crosslinked polymer containing 1 mole% copolymerized 9,10-dihydroxystearic acid. Scanning electron microscopy of explanted devices shown in Figure 10 reveal an erosion process (Heller, 1985) confined predominantly to the outer surface of the cylindrical devices.

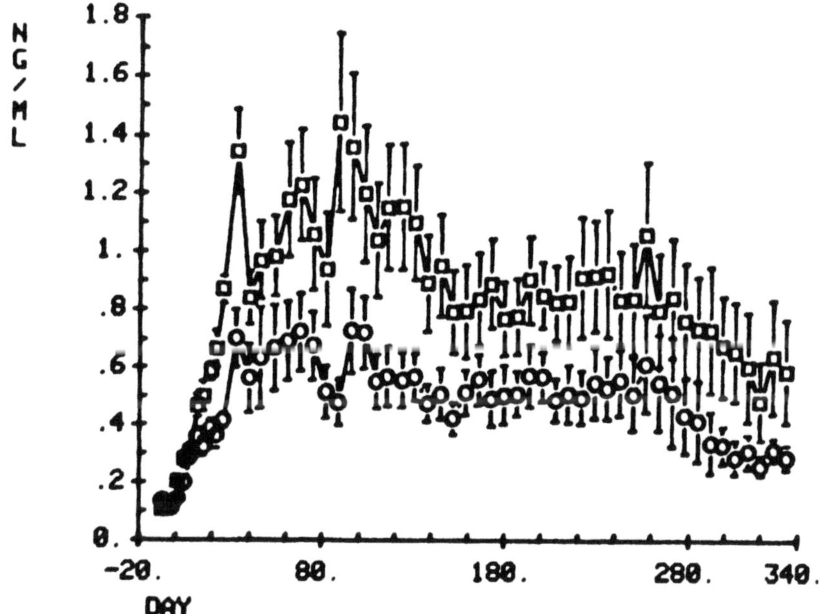

Figure 9. Daily rabbit blood plasma levels of levonorgestrel from crosslinked poly(ortho ester) rods 2.4 x 20 mm formed from a diketene acetal, 3-methyl-1,5-pentanediol 1,2,6-hexanetriol and 1 mole % copolymerized dihydroxystearic acid containing 30 wt % levonorgestrel and 7 wt % $Mg(OH)_2$ ○ device/rabbit □ 2 devices/rabbit

The third surface-eroding polymer system are polyanhydrides. Polyanhydrides were first prepared as potential textile fibers (Hill and Carothers, 1932), but were abandoned due to poor hydrolytic stability. However, it was also recognized that aromatic polyanhydrides are relatively stable, and their stability has been attributed to the crystalline nature of the polymer (Conix, 1958).

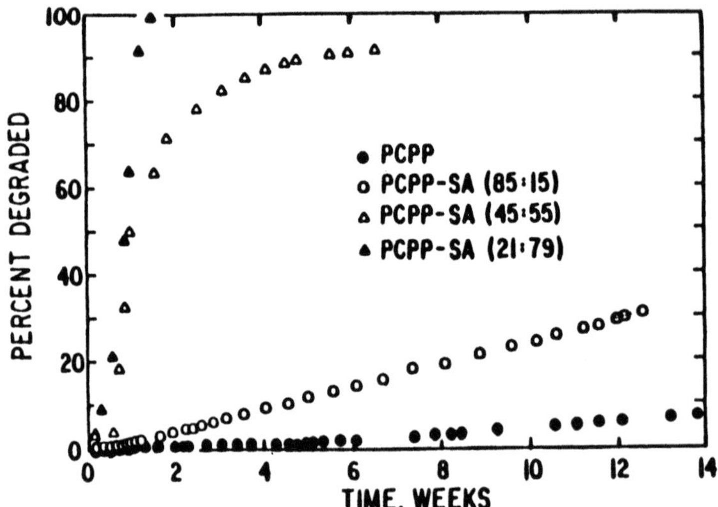

Figure 10. Degradation profiles of compression molded poly bis(p-carboxyphenoxy) propane anhydride and its copolymers with sebacic acid in 0.1 M pH 7.4 phosphate buffer at 37°C. Reprinted with permission from Leong KW, Brott BC, Langer R (1985). Bioerodible polyanhydrides as drug carrier matrices I: Characterization, degradation and release characteristics. J. Biomed. Mater. Res. 19: 941-955

Polyanhydrides formed from aliphatic and aromatic diacids are currently being investigated as a surface eroding system for the delivery of incorporated therapeutic agents, and results of in vitro erosion studies are shown in Figure 11 (Leong, Brott, and Langer, 1985). Clearly, incorporation of an aliphatic segment into the polymer has a significant effect on rate of erosion, and variations in the amount of aliphatic segments relative to the aromatic segments provide a means of varying erosion times within a very wide range. Because the polymer degrades to dicarboxylic acids no toxicological difficulties are anticipated. However, due to the high reactivity of the anhydride linkage, care must be taken during fabrication of devices to avoid reactions between the anhydride linkage and reactive groups such as amines or hydroxyls in the incorporated therapeutic agent.

REFERENCES

Baker RW, Lonsdale HK (1974) Controlled release: mechanism and rates. In: Tanquary AC, Lacey RE, (eds): Controlled release of biologically active agents. Plenum Press, New York; pp 15-71

Beck LR, Ramos RA, Flowers CE Jr., Lopez GZ, Lewis DH, Cowsar DR (1981) Clinical evaluation of injectable biodegradable contraceptive systems. Am. J. Obstet. Gynecol. 140:799-806

Beck LR, Flowers CE Jr., Pope VZ, Wilborn WH, Tice TR (1983) Clinical evaluation of an improved injectable microcapsule contraceptive system. Am. J. Obstet. Gynecol. 147:815-821

Conix A (1958) Aromatic polyanhydrides, a new class of high melting fiber-forming polymers. J. Polymer Sci. 29:343-353

Frazza EJ, Schmitt EE (1971) A new absorbable suture. J. Biomed. Mater. Res. Symp. 1: 43-58

Heller J, Baker RW, Gale RM, Rodin JO (1978) Controlled drug release by polymer dissolution I. Partial esters of maleic anhydride copolymers. Properties and theory. J. Appl. Polymer Sci. 22:1991-2009

Heller J (1980) Controlled release of biologically active compounds from bioerodible polymers. Biomaterials 1:51-57

Heller J, Penhale DWH, Helwing RF (1980) Preparation of poly(ortho esters) by the reaction of ketene acetals and polyols. J. Polymer Sci., Polymer Lett. Ed. 18:619-624

Heller J (1984) Biodegradable polymers in controlled drug delivery. CRC Critical Reviews in Therap. Drug Carrier Syst. 1:39-90

Heller J, Penhale DWH, Fritzinger BK, Ng SY (1984) Controlled release of contraceptive agents from poly(ortho esters). In: Zatuchni GK, Goldsmith A, Shelton JD, Sciarra J (eds): Long acting contraceptive delivery systems. Harper and Row, Philadelphia; pp 113-128

Heller J (1985) Controlled drug release from poly(ortho esters) - a surface eroding polymer. J. Controlled Release 2:167-177

Heller J, Fritzinger BK, Ng SY, and Penhale DWH (1985) In vitro and in vivo release of levonorgestrel from crosslinked poly(ortho esters) II crosslinked polymers. J. Controlled Release 1:233-238

Heller J, Penhale DWH, Fritzinger BK, Ng SY (1987) The effect of copolymerized 9,10-dihydroxystearic acid on erosion rates of poly(ortho esters). J. Controlled Release, in press

Higuchi T (1961) Rates of release of medicaments from ointment bases containing drugs in suspension. J. Pharm. Sci. 50:874-875

Hill JW, Carothers WC (1932) Studies of polymerization and ring formation XIV. A linear superpolyanhydride and a cyclic dimeric anhydride from sebacic acid. J. Am. Chem. Soc. 54:1569-1579

Hsieh DST, Rhine WD, Langer R (1983) Zero-order controlled release polymer matrices for micro- and macromolecules. J. Pharm. Sci. 72:17-22

Kulkarni RK, Pani KC, Neuman C, Leonard F (1966) Polylactic acid for surgical implants. Arch. Surg. 93:839-843

Langer R, Peppas N (1983) Chemical and physical structure of polymers as carriers for controlled release of bioactive agents: a review. Rev. Macromol. Chem. Phys. C23: 61-126

Lee PI (1985) Kinetics of drug release from hydrogel matrices. J. Controlled Release 2:277-288

Leong KW, Brott BC, Langer R (1985) Bioerodible polyanhydrides as drug-carrier matrices I: characterization, degradation, and release characteristics. J. Biomed. Mater. Res. 19:941-955

Sparer RV, Shih C, Ringeisen CD, Himmelstein KJ (1984) Controlled release from erodible poly(ortho ester) drug delivery systems. J. Controlled Release 1:23-32

CONCLUDING REMARKS

A broad spectrum has been treated during this two-day International Symposium on ophthalmic drug delivery, reaching from biopharmaceutical to technological and clinical domains. Furthermore, new or improved ocular drug delivery systems were observed in extenso, sometimes employing clever tests in vitro but especially in vivo on animals (rabbits, cats, monkeys etc.). Another aspect dealt with sustained and controlled drug release kinetics with various simple *and* sophisticated dosage forms or therapeutic systems.

An additional group of subjects discussed rôle and influence of the excipients or carriers of resin matrixes, polymers, hydrophilic colloidal systems with anionic and kationic surfactants, lenses, inserts and other devices.

No doubt, clarification and progress could be clearly recognized and this International Symposium entirely fulfilled its purpose.

Nevertheless, some creative criticism should not be omitted. In vitro models, even cell cultures, in vivo models of animal studies on a rabbit, monkey or cat, are not representative for humans. Such investigation can offer us basic ideas, trends, tendencies, suggestions, hopes etc. but will never be the final answer to an ocular problem. Only clinical studies on man, for the sake of the patient, if possible on a double blind base or on other scientifically accepted methods can serve to decide whether a delivery system proves to be adequate or not and whether research should advance into this or that direction. For ophthalmic drug delivery systems clinical studies are essential, and such a procedure is an absolute necessity or *conditio sine qua non* to achieve optimal results.

This fact is also one of the main reasons to intensify the close collaboration between physicians and pharmacists, ophthalmologists and drug designers. An excellent start has been made at this Symposium, and the collaboration between medicine and pharmacy was promising. This fruitful co-operation should even be improved in the future.

Outlook: The International participants of this Ophthalmic Drug Delivery Symposium were highly interested to learn:

- how ophthalmic drug delivery will develop;
- which therapeutic systems will be the forms of the future and
- what are the trends in drug delivery systems on, into and through the eye, i.e. epi-, endo- and maybe diaocular delivery.

The future ophthalmic delivery trends will no doubt go into the following directions:

1) Optimization of the classical drug design.

Better knowledge of our actual ocular pharmaca and excipients concerning biologic and physico-chemical properties as pH, pK-values, partition-, diffusion-, penetration-, and permeation coefficients is needed. These physico-chemical data should not only be known for the macroenvironment but also on the cellular level. This field lacks attention in many respects, is often neglected, yet has been skimmed during this Symposium.

2) Development of ophthalmic prodrugs.

Chemically modified drug in form of prodrug with distinct physico-chemical properties and similar biological activities have a chance in the near future. Prodrugs are pre-steps of pharmaca which are not active but may liberate the active drug during or after application in a controlled manner.

3) New ophthalmic drug design.

Another tendency of research should be the development of new drugs against the most embarassing diseases discussed, such as glaucoma, cataract, dry eye syndrome etc. Such drugs have *not* been debated but could well be one of our future targets in research.

4) Better drug delivery systems.

Hydrogels: the design of hydrogels which increase their viscosity instantaneously after medication, liberate the drug according to a desired *rate of release* and finally biodegrade the hydrogel with all the other excipients of the system.

Ultrafine colloidal vesicles or particles with biodegradable macromolecules and no, or a minimum of, adjuvants would be highly desirable as improved micro- and nanocapsules, liposomes and eye-friendly, non-irritating pharmacosomes. Furthermore, biodegradable inserts and lamellas which do not create any serious interactions would be badly wanted.

The problem of sophisticated microdevices or controlled ocular drug delivery without serious irritations is probably one of the most urgent research fields to be observed in ocular drug delivery design.

5) Safety of ophthalmic drug delivery systems.

All further developments and trends must respect the physiology of our ophthalmic drug delivery systems.

Acute, subacute and chronic toxicity studies as well as local or systemic irritation should in future be studied more profoundly. Furthermore, side-reactions of immunobiologic, allergic, anaphylactic genesis must expressly be excluded completely because safety of the eye medication is one of the main requirements in ophthalmic therapy.

I sometimes wonder if our excipients used, the resins, the polymers, the surfactants, the preservatives, the containers and devices are really safe. I often doubt that one considers the enzymatic attack on these materials:

- the formation of metabolisation in the eye;
- the rest-monomer content of many drug delivery systems, lenses, inserts, devices etc.;
- the excipients which are not safe. Let us only think of a softener such as polyethyleneglycols;
- preservatives as aromatic alcohols and
- the lack of sterility due to primary, secondary or tertiary contamination.

All these reflections presented now show quite clearly that there is not only a need but a necessity to go on with our scientific eye medication activities and with the exchange of opinions because progress is very slow. Therefore, I warmly recommend to continue with such successful symposia, not to loiter, nor rest or sleep on laurels but go on and try to make a tradition of this so excellently organized International Symposium on Ophthalmic Drug Delivery.

P. Speiser

SUBJECT INDEX

ERRATA

Ophthalmic Drug Delivery. Biopharmaceutical, Technological and Clinical Aspects.
M.F. Saettone, M. Bucci, P. Speiser (eds)

On the cover and at the bottom of the first page of each chapter: "M.S. Saettone, G. Bucci, P. Speiser" please read "M.F. Saettone, M. Bucci, P. Speiser".
The Publishers wish to apologise to the reader.

GPSR Compliance
The European Union's (EU) General Product Safety Regulation (GPSR) is a set of rules that requires consumer products to be safe and our obligations to ensure this.

If you have any concerns about our products, you can contact us on

ProductSafety@springernature.com

In case Publisher is established outside the EU, the EU authorized representative is:

Springer Nature Customer Service Center GmbH
Europaplatz 3
69115 Heidelberg, Germany

www.ingramcontent.com/pod-product-compliance
Ingram Content Group UK Ltd.
Pitfield, Milton Keynes, MK11 3LW, UK
UKHW051126260726
13967UKWH00010B/2897